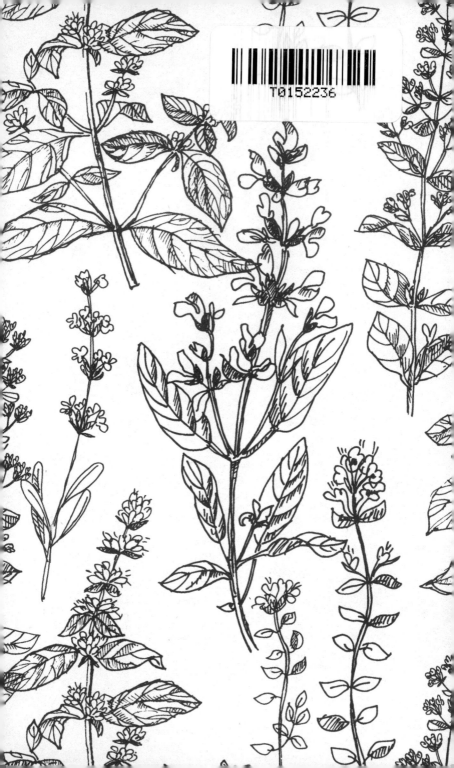

The
Herbal
Healing
Handbook

The Herbal Healing Handbook

How to Use Plants, Essential Oils and Aromatherapy as Natural Remedies

Cerridwen Greenleaf

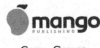

CORAL GABLES

Disclaimer: This book is not intended as a substitute for the medical advice of physicians. The reader should regularly consult a physician in matters relating to his/her health and particularly with respect to any symptoms that may require diagnosis or medical attention.

The Herbal Healing Handbook: How to Use Plants, Essential Oils and Aromatherapy as Natural Remedies

Library of Congress Cataloging-in-Publication number: 2020946331
ISBN: (print) 978-1-63353-714-9 , (ebook) 978-1-63353-715-6
BISAC category code: HEA009000, HEALTH & FITNESS / Healing

Printed in the United States of America

This book is for all the wise women healers who came before me. We are only here because of you.

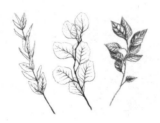

"The brilliance of the seas has flashed forth. The dawn of the blessing has arisen. What IS this ancient wisdom? The source of these living waters is in your head and in your eyes."

—Rumi

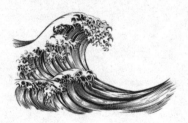

Table of Contents

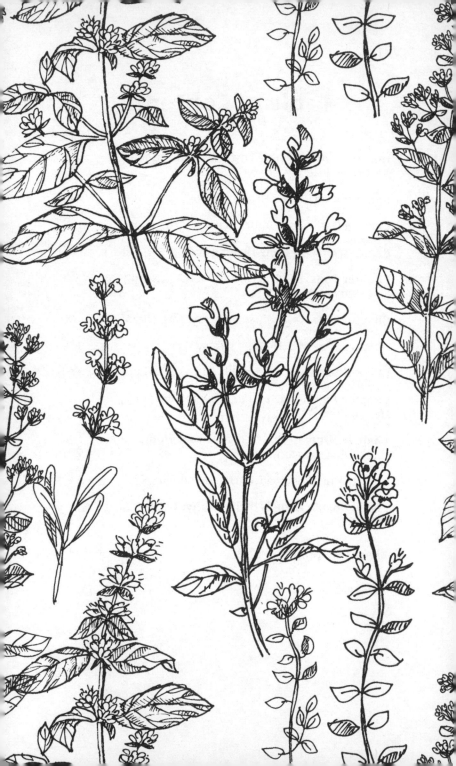

INTRODUCTION

How We Lost Our Connection to Nature and How We Can Get It Back

On woodland walks, my Aunt Edie pointed out nettles, wild mint, Queen Anne's Lace, and other herbs which grew by creek beds near my home. We picked, steeped, and sipped concoctions we made together as she imparted her homely wisdom. Little did I know at the time I was being gently schooled as an apprentice kitchen witch. Lately, I have been called upon to craft spells for peace of mind; so many of us are overwhelmed due to the fragmented lifestyles requiring long hours at work, zillions of emails, texts, tweets, and all the demands that don't stop coming.

How often do you see a panicky pagan or stressed out herbalist? Rarely, I assure you.

We all have to keep pace with the modern world, but our connection to the earth and the cycles of nature help maintain balance and harmony, despite the hurly-burly of these tech-driven times. This chapter is aimed at conjuring wellness so you can stay centered, grounded, and healthy. When our grandmothers and elders who came before us tended cuts, bruises, colds, flus, fevers, and other illnesses their family suffered, they didn't have a corner drugstore. Instead, these wise women relied on simple wisdom, common sense, and pantries well-stocked with herbal remedies. These preparations were made from plants that grew in the kitchen garden or wild weeds gathered in the fields and woods surrounding their homes. This stash of kitchen cupboard cures combines the wisdom of our elders with a modern sensibility. Yes, you will save money, but more importantly, you will begin to learn what works for you and master the art of self-care as you bring much comfort to your loved ones.

CHAPTER ONE

Major Healing Herbs: Mother Nature's Guide to Good Health

Do you refresh with sprigs of mint or sip chamomile tea regularly? Do you purify your space with sage? Are rosemary, mint, and lavender favorites in your sachets and teas? Think of all the herbs and plants you love and use often, then begin researching their upkeep and care. Make sure to research your planting zone so you sort out the optimal climate conditions to nurture your plants and herbs. Once you have planned your plantings, infuse your plot with magical intention. Keep careful track of your progress in your herbal journal. As you grow in experience and expertise, so will the healing power of your plot.

Remember to research plants and herbs that can be toxic or poisonous to ensure the safety of children or our canine and feline friends. Most of the flower power handed down to us is excellent for magical workings, but not at all appropriate for tea, edibles, or such. Make sure visiting children stay far away from wisteria, rhododendron, lily of the valley, Narcissus, foxglove, larkspur, hydrangea, and oleander. They are beautiful but deadly—literally.

A Note About Materials

When you make herbal preparations, ideally avoid using plastic cups or nonstick-coated pots to steep and simmer your plant medicines (although plastic measuring spoons should not be harmful). Aluminum is likewise not favored by herbalists. An ideal pot in which to simmer medicinal roots and barks will be made of either Pyrex or steel; ceramics that are food safe should be fine for preparing infusions, whether in a teapot or cup. (You may want to acquire a *small* saucepan to simmer up individually tailored potions, as well as perhaps also a larger pot for brews needed in quantity.) Whether you are simmering barks and roots or infusing leaves and flowers, you will need a lid to cover your pot or cup so that the volatile essences that give medicinal herbs their healing power do not dissipate into the air.

Twenty-Two Healing Herbs: Mother Nature's Medicine Cabinet

Ashwagandha (*Withania somnifera*)

Gently simmer one tablespoon of dried and minced ashwagandha root in one cup of water for eight to ten minutes. Strain and sip once or twice a day as a rejuvenating pick-me-up, anti-inflammatory, anxiety reducer, and immunity tonic.

Black Cohosh (*Actaea racemosa*)

Make a tincture or use the flower essence method in this book and take twenty to forty drops three times a day to relieve menstrual cramps and arthritic pain. Black cohosh can also help perimenopausal and menopausal symptoms.

Calendula (*Calendula officinalis*)

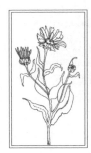 Boil one cup of water and pour over two teaspoons of calendula petals. Steep this for eight to ten minutes and strain. Once it has cooled enough, you can drink it as a tea, use it as a mouthwash, or gargle with it to reduce any swelling of the mouth or throat. If you make an ointment with calendula, apply it to your skin three times during the day and it will calm irritation.

This commonly used herbal aid is popular for relief of gastrointestinal issues including oral and throat inflammation. It can also be made into a salve to heal the skin and soothe rashes, itching, irritation, and wounds. Remember that any herb can be made into a salve following the Calming Balm: Bay Leaf recipe in Chapter Four. Your family will probably request the comfort of the calendula salve often, so keep it handy.

Catnip (*Nepeta cataria*)

Dry a palmful of catnip leaves and allow them to steep in a cup of boiling water for five minutes, then strain as you would any loose tea. Honey helps even more, and a cup or two of catnip tea per day will have

you in fine fettle, relaxed, and ready. This herb is not just for kitties! We humans can also benefit from it as a remedy for upset tummies as well as a way to diminish worry, anxiety, and nervous tension.

Cranberry (*Vaccinium macrocarpon*)

How many times did your mom tell you to drink your (usually unsweetened) cranberry juice? Turns out she was right on both counts as straight cranberry juice is very good for bladder health and benefits men's prostates; two half cups a day, mom's orders!

Echinacea (*Echinacea spp.*)

Every herb store or organic grocer will have dried echinacea root for fighting colds and negating respiratory infections. Just mince by the teaspoon and simmer low covered in two cups of boiling water. Sweeten to taste and drink at least a couple of cups a day, echinacea also makes an excellent tincture you can make by following the how-tos herein. It is an amazing immune booster, too!

Elderberry (*Sambucus nigra, S. canadensis*)

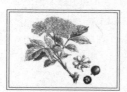 This time-tested medicinal has long been used for guarding against colds and flu. Elderberry flowers have been valued as a tonic for fever for centuries; such fruit

extracts have been proven to be noteworthy antivirals, especially to support immunity. Two teaspoons of dried flowers and a cup of boiling water three times a day does the trick. Sweeten with local honey to taste. Or consider cultivating elderberry and making a syrup.

Local Honey Heals!

Why local? Here's why. Allergies can exacerbate any cold or respiratory illness. Many who suffer seasonal allergies have found local, raw honey to be wonderfully helpful as it desensitizes them to the flora that trigger their allergic reaction. Twice as sweet!

Garlic (*Allium sativum*)

We have all heard that the Chinese praise garlic for health benefits. It is a powerful antimicrobial, often employed to combat colds, ease sinus congestion, and stave off digestive problems that accompany traveling. It has even been shown that regular use can help gently lower blood pressure. One to two fresh cloves daily are the dose.

Ginger (*Zingiber officinale*)

From tummy troubles to colds and flus, ginger is beloved for its curative powers. Any greengrocer or herbal apothecary will have plenty or ginger root in stock, and you should always have some around. When anyone in your family feels nauseous or senses a cold or fever coming, slice and mince a tablespoon of the root into two cups of hot water and simmer it low covered for tea.

Sweeten to taste and drink twice a day for a surprisingly swift end to your suffering. It also makes a wonderful spicy iced tea when cooled, though for a respiratory or tummy bug, drink it comfortably warm.

Ginseng (*Panax quinquefolius*; *P. ginseng*)

Many people rely upon ginseng to relieve and avert mental and physical fatigue. This herb has been shown to reduce the occurrence and acuteness of colds. Some even claim it can help with issues of male virility. It can help to light the fire of vitality within your body; for this reason, if you have spells of feeling *too* warm, limit your intake of ginseng. Either dried or fresh will do, three times a day simmered in a cup of freshly boiled water for eight to ten minutes. (Note that Siberian "ginseng" is a different plant entirely and is in fact a distinct species from another plant family, *Eleutherococcus senticocus*; it is also useful as a nutritive and grounding adaptogen, but should not be confused with Asian or American ginseng!)

Hibiscus (*Hibiscus sabdariffa*)

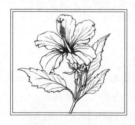

Beloved for the heavenly sweet perfume of its flowers, hibiscus is also a powerful diuretic and can lower blood pressure. As if that is not enough, it can also help sore throats and colds. Similarly to other herbal applications, steeping a tablespoon of the dried flowers in a cup of freshly boiled water for ten minutes and drinking this infusion twice a day is the desired treatment.

Hops (*Humulus lupulus*)

As we all know, hops are used for beer-making and excel as a tincture used as a sleeping aid and stress-reliever. Women healers also claim it is very useful to calm hot flashes in menopause. The ideal dosage is forty drops before sleep. It is said it can help anxiety. Lower your dose if you wake up extra sleepy in the morning after using hops.

Kava (*Piper methysticum*)

This root is also said to be highly effective as a muscle relaxer and for reducing anxiety. Kava can be handled the same as ginger, with one tablespoon of minced root or dried root simmered low and taken as tea. I recommend seeing how it affects you before you raise the dose to two or three cups of tea per day, which is recommended. If you take it as a supplement, when considering taking more than 250 mg. per day (a fraction of the weight of a US penny) or for longer than a week, make sure you are under the care of a qualified health professional. As with many, many powerful remedies, if you take it *all* the time without breaks, it won't work anymore right when you need it most.

Licorice (*Glycyrrhiza glabra*)

This revered candy classic is also a wonderful anti-inflammatory which relieves the discomfort of colds in the sinuses. It can soothe sore throats and coughs and is a curative for gastrointestinal issues. Treat licorice root exactly as you would ginger with one minced teaspoon of fresh or dried simmered low covered in one cup of water twice a day to make a naturally sweet tea. Also, you can add licorice root to other herbal teas as it will sweeten them, besides adding its medicinal virtues, which tend to combine well with those of many other basic remedies.

Marshmallow (*Althaea officinalis*)

While it may seem like this is another "candy as medicine," marshmallow is a time-tested *plant* long employed in field medicine rather than a sugary pillow. It is highly valued as it contains a lot of mucilage, the same substance which coats our mouth and throat as well as the stomach and gut. Minced fresh, dried root, or the leaves are equally healing in quarter cup quantities; an infusion of the leaves may be drunk after it has steeped for four hours covered. Strain out the stems and drink hot, cool, sweetened, or however you like this gentle herb. If you choose marshmallow root, simmer low covered for twenty minutes, then let cool; the brew may be taken at any temperature you prefer.

Milk Thistle (*Silybum manianum*)

Healers love milk thistle for its ability to protect the liver from toxins, harsh medicines, alcohol, and unseen environmental pollutants. It can be obtained as either an extract or in standardized capsules at any health food store or upscale grocery or pharmacy. There is some evidence it can also help heal the kidneys. If you want to get the most bang for your buck, find a source of organic milk thistle *seed*, then thoroughly clean out a coffee grinder as the seeds must be broken open in order to be bioavailable via digestion. The milk thistle seeds need not be ground to powder; instead, grind them small enough that when sprinkled on a soup, stew, or salad it isn't too chewy—their taste is pleasant. A tablespoon or two a day can be a real lifesaver!

Mullein (*Verbascum Thapsus*)

Here is an herbalist's favorite for healing any respiratory ailment involving congestion, coughs, sore throats, and supporting lung function and clear breathing. Take one heaping tablespoon of the leaves and steep in one cup of boiling water covered for no more than ten minutes. Once you take mullein as a tea, you'll feel better soon. Mullein flowers infused in oil are also used to aid earaches.

Nettle (*Urtica dioica*)

Nettle has been used as a healer for untold centuries; it relieves allergies, it is an immune booster, and it can even help with a distended prostate. It is also a superfood and beloved for its nutrients. If you are working with fresh nettles, wear gloves to avoid the stinging. Cooking or drying removes any irritant. Any herb or health food store will have dried nettle both in bulk and capsule form. Make nettle tea by steeping two teaspoons of leaves for ten minutes covered or take the capsules in recommended doses of 300 to 500 mg twice a day.

Sage (*Salvia officinalis*)

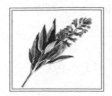 We know sage is great for as a smudge or incense for clearing spaces as well as a savory for soups, roasts, dressing, stews, and much more, but it is also a highly regarded treatment at European spas for sweating, menopause, hot flashes,

night sweats and accompanying discomfort. It is also an excellent remedy for colds, coughs, and sore throats. Simply make sage tea with one teaspoon of the dried leaves which you can drink or gargle to amend a sore throat.

Note: Pregnant women should not use this.

Slippery Elm Bark (*Ulmus rubra*)

Slippery Elm Bark has even been approved by the FDA as a remedy for the irritation of sore throats and other sighs of an impending cold, including coughs. This herbal can also help with stomach upset and help with heartburn. A powdered version of the bark can easily be obtained at any health food store or upscale greengrocer, which can be made into a tea; use one to two teaspoons of the powdered bark, and you can drink it twice a day.

St. John's Wort (*Hypericum perforatum*)

This is one of the most relied-upon of all herbal treatments for mild to moderate depression, PMS, perimenopause symptoms, and general immune and mood boosting, It is so popular now that you can find the extract in capsules at most pharmacies, grocers, herbal supply stores, and the like. Take three to six hundred milligrams per day to brighten your days. You can also find St. John's Wort as a tincture if you prefer a liquid extract.

Thyme (*Thymus vulgaris*)

Thyme has so much to offer, including relief for colds, coughs, and congestion; above all, it is an antimicrobial and antispasmodic. One cup of tea made from a teaspoon of dried thyme leaves steeped in boiling water will bring much healing energy to you and your family.

Plenty of Thyme—An Herb for Physical and Spiritual Strength

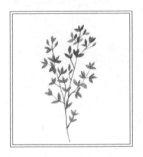 You could say that thyme is a classic herb, so much so that the venerables, Virgil and Pliny, sang the praises of this medicinal mint relative over two thousand years ago. While thyme loves Mediterranean weather, it can grow elsewhere from seeds and cuttings. Good for the stomach and especially effective as respiratory relief, thyme induces sweats to remove toxins and reduce fever. Thyme honey tea is truly a sweet way to make the medicine go down, so much so you will find you drink it even when hale and hearty. Thyme is also a culinary plant, making it a delightful additive to savory dishes. When I lived in a warmer clime about ten years ago, I planted wooly thyme in among the flagstones of my front yard and let it spread as much as possible. By the hour when I came home from work, the sunny eighty-plus degree sunny weather

had warmed the thyme, creating a perfumed walkway; coming home was a heavenly experience.

It has been believed for centuries that thyme brings courage and both inner and physical strength. Even when you are facing seemingly insurmountable odds, spells and smudging featuring thyme can get you on track and bring you to your goal. I think the greatest of all aspects of thyme is to rid your home and family of melancholy and overcome despair after extreme difficulty and loss. If your loved ones have experienced a catastrophe, try thyme for rituals of magic and restitution. I have no doubt that practitioners of green witchery will be singing the praises of thyme for at least two thousand more years.

Sleepy Thyme

This herb improves your quality of sleep; gather and dry thyme it to use in sachets so the divine fragrance freshens linens and laundry. A little bag of this dried thyme tucked in your pillowcase makes for sweeter sleep. As if all that is not enough, the plant itself also repels bugs and pests but attracts honeybees! As we all know, deep sleep is a great healer.

Lemon Balm Soothes Those Aches and Pains (Including Heartbreak)

Balm also goes by the equally lovely Latinate name *Melissa. From Greco-Roman times,* this relative of the mint family has been held to be a significant medicinal. You can grow lemon balm with ease from seed packets in almost any kind of soil, but it likes shade in the afternoon to prevent wilting. This is one of the happy plants that will "volunteer" to spread in your garden, and it can be used in your home to bring love to you and to heal after a breakup or divorce. It can also be employed as an aphrodisiac. Infusions and teas made from lemon balm make good on the offer the name implies as it can soothe the heart and any lingering upset, blue moods, or aches and pains from trauma, both physical and emotional. I suggest we all grow as much as possible and let some go to seed for those new plants that will pop up in unexpected places in your herb garden. An herbalist never complains about a plentitude of balm; anyone who makes much use of lemon balm in brews and cookery will enjoy an abundance of love.

Cheer Up with Chives

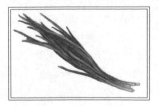
Allium, also known as chives, is blessedly easy plant to grow anywhere and everywhere— on the kitchen windowsill or in the garden patch. A

member of the onion family, this is a lovely case where the entire plant—bulb, leaves, and flowers—can be eaten. Plant the bulbs six inches apart, water them, and you can pretty much ignore them after that as all they require is water. A plus is that this relative of onion has insect repellent properties, so you can plant rows of this beside veggies and fruits and the bugs will stay away. They propagate quickly, so you can dig up mature bulbs, separate them, and replant them. One tip to remember is that chives do lose their flavor when dried, so use them fresh. The flowers are a lovely surprise to add to salads for their edible beauty, and many a kitchen gardener uses chives in all manner of dishes as it is good for weight management and is a plant of protection for both home and garden. Chives were used by healers of old in amulets to ward off evil spirits and mischievous fairy folk. Fresh cut bunches were also hung beside the sickbed to speed healing, especially for children. If you see a home surrounded by rows of allium, you know they hold to the "old ways."

Basil Bliss

This sweet tasting herb is excellent in savory dishes. Basil truly grows like a weed, and you should cultivate it right on the kitchen windowsill so you can snip basil leaves to add to your Thai or Italian-inspired dishes. Give your basil plants plenty of sun and lots of water and you will reap a mighty bounty to share with the neighbors. Old wives and hedge witches claim basil protects while it brings prosperity and happiness to any gardener's home. Basil helps steady the mind, brings happiness, love, peace, and money, and even protects against insanity. (What more can you want?) The benefits of this plant are as plentiful as the plant itself; it can be used for manifesting and attracting love and on the highest vibrational level for abetting psychic abilities, even astral projection.

Edible Flowers

Organic pesticide-free posies are tasty additions to salads, cake décor, and even savories such as fried squash blossoms. Florals add a stunning beauty to any dish. Grab your basket and add a bouquet to your culinary creations: impatiens, marigold, gladiola, daylily, cornflower, daisy, carnation, and viola. My favorites are peppery, fresh-flavored nasturtiums, which are so easy to grow, have a lovely aroma, and their yellow, red, and orange-bright blooms are the color of happiness.

Coltsfoot Cures Coughs

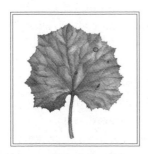

Coltsfoot, also called Butterbur, is so named for the leaf's resemblance to a horse's hoof. Viewed as a weed, except by those who know, this spiky flowering plant grows wild along creeks, wetlands, or loamy fields. *Tussilago*, its Latinate botanical name, means "cough dispeller," and this is a powerful aid to those with asthma or bronchial conditions and is very good medicine for colds and flu. In folklore, young maidens would use the leaves in a simple spell to see their future husband off in the distance galloping toward her. Truly knowledgeable hedge healers have a herd of coltsfoot in the shadiest, dampest part of their property. Coltsfoot's medicinal mojo can be unleashed by infusing its leaves and/or flowers as a steeped tea. It is also commonly used as an ingredient in non-tobacco smoking blends; though naturally smoking of any sort is stressful to the lungs, if someone is determined to smoke in any case, smoking a little coltsfoot is thought to be a lung tonic.

Angelica, the Digestive of the Heavens

Angelica, said to first bloom on the Archangel Michael's name day, is part of the carrot family and is a tall, hollow-stemmed plant with umbrella-shaped clusters of pale white flowers, tinged with green. Candying the stalks in sugar was an old-fashioned favorite; angelica was also traditionally used to cure colds and relieve coughs. Nowadays, seeds are used to make chartreuse, a digestive and uniquely tasty liqueur. This heavenly guardian flower is a protector, as one might expect for a plant associated with archangels, and it is used to reverse curses, break hexes, and fend off negative energies. An angelica root, dried and cured, is a traditional talisman that can be carried in your pocket or in an amulet to bring long life. Many a wise woman has used angelica leaves in baths and rituals to rid a household of dark spirits. If the bad energy is intense, burn the angelica leaves with frankincense to exorcise it from your space. While you are protecting yourself and your home from negativity during this angelica smudging session, you will also experience heightened psychism. Pay close attention to your dreams after this; important messages will come through.

Herbal Amulets: Handmade Gifts of Caring and Curing

You will experience years of enjoyment from tending your garden, as Voltaire taught us in his masterpiece, *Candide*. You can share that pleasure with your friends and those you love by giving gifts from your garden. Your good intentions will be returned many times over. I keep a stock of small muslin drawstring bags for creating amulets. If you are a crafty person, you can make the bags, too, sewing them by hand before stuffing the dried herbs inside.

- For courage and strength of heart: Mullein or borage

- For good cheer: Nettle or yarrow

- For fellow witches: Ivy, broomstraw, and maidenhair fern

- For safe travels: Comfrey

- For fertility: Cyclamen or mistletoe

- For protection from deceit: Snapdragon

- For good health: Rue

- For success: Woodruff

- For strength: Mugwort

❧ For youthful looks: An acorn

Amulets should be kept on your person at all times, either in a pocket, in your purse or book bag, or on a string around your neck.

Daisy and Echinacea: Healing the Heart and Body

This faithful flower's name is derived from the Anglo-Saxon *daeges eage*, "day's eye," since it closes in the evening. The daisy has been used in one of the oldest of love charms. To know if your true love will return, take a daisy and intone, "He loves me, he loves me not" until the last petal is plucked, and the answer will be revealed. This flower is not just a boon for romance, however; it also useful in herbal medicine for aches, bruises, wounds, inflammation, and soothing eye baths. As a flower remedy, it is quite helpful with exhaustion and is a highly regarded remedy in homeopathy. Echinacea, also known as purple coneflower, is a member of the daisy family that has become wildly popular as a healer for colds and as a powerful immune booster; it both increases your T cell count and helps to fight off illnesses both minor and major. Echinacea is an herb of abundance that attracts abundant prosperity, but it can also be used in magic workings to amplify the power.

Rosemary Restores You

Rosemary is another of the herbs that thrive best in warm Mediterranean climes but can weather the cold. Tough to grow from seed, cuttings are an easier way to start your row of rosemary plants in your garden. Pots of this bushy plant can enjoy being outdoors in spring and summer and then come in from the cold to a sheltered porch or inside by a sunny window. As a bonus, it requires little water. Rosemary is fantastic as a seasoning for potatoes or roast chicken and makes any Sunday supper taste better and brighter. You can pinch off the aromatic needles to dress plates or sprinkle into soups and stews. Beyond all of what it can do to enhance your cookery, this is a primary plant for rejuvenation. It is prized for how it restores after lingering illness; elixirs and essential oils made from rosemary stimulate, raise mental alertness, and energize as they comfort. In Greco-Roman times, rosemary was believed to help the memory. An excellent kitchen witchery practice is to take dried or fresh rosemary and add it to a steam for an easy infusion where it aids breathing, muscle aches, and anxiety. You can accomplish the same by adding rosemary to a hot bath, either in a fresh sprig or wrapped in a little cheesecloth to keep the rosemary from scattering. Lie back and relax, remembering happy times in your life and those that lie right ahead of you.

The Scent of Sheer Joy

Lavender is blessedly easy to grow as it is a shrubby plant of Mediterranean origins. It is prized for its lovely scent and is a very powerful healing plant with many other properties: it is used for making teas and tisanes, infusing into honey, and many other practical uses. It can even prosper in dry and drought-prone areas, so make sure your kitchen garden has at least one of the hardy varieties of lavender so you can dry bundles to use in your spellwork as well as in your recipes.

Lavender Aromatherapy: The Sweet Smell of Serenity

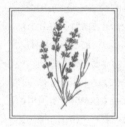

The time you take to restore yourself is precious. Morning is the optimal time to perform a self-blessing, which will help you maintain both your physical health and provide an emotional boost. Today, lavender oil is the most popular essential oil the world over, but the benefits of lavender were actually discovered over three thousand years ago. Because of its deeply powerful calming and soothing effect as well as antioxidant, antimicrobial, sedative, tranquilizing, and antidepressive properties, lavender oil is simply wonderful—even the scent brings joy. When King Tut's tomb in Egypt was opened in 1923, a faint perfume of lavender remained after three thousand years. In the Bible, lavender was beloved for anointing and healing. Lavender, let us count the ways we love you:

➳ Anxiety reduction and lessening emotional stress

➳ Protection against diabetes

- Improved brain function
- Healing burns and wounds
- Better sleep
- Brightens skin health and circulation
- Slows down aging with powerful antioxidants
- Pain relief
- Alleviate headaches

Find Your Celestial Essence: Twelve Floral Healers for Each Sign of the Zodiac

Floral waters and flower essentials express emotional benefits differently, and each flower has a unique and special healing application. As we can tell from the mass popularity of Bach's Rescue Remedy, flowers work wonderfully to abet emotional health, mental centeredness, and positivity. The specific of these curatives can be pretty direct. For example, the flower impatiens helps those who struggle with impatience. Magical, right? Below you'll find one flower essence for each of the twelve signs. Read yours and learn what can work for you:

Aries: Impatiens Renewal for Rams

 High energy Aries often race forward as they blaze new trails. Patience is not their strong suit. When the going gets tough, they just race forward, never stopping,

However, this can also be a major source of undue stress and strain; try impatiens flower essence and you'll discover a wellspring of fortitude.

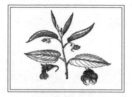

Impatiens

Taurus: Chestnut Bud Benefits for Bulls

Home, prosperity, and security loving Taureans prefer safe harbor and no surprises. This routinized life can lead to getting into a bit of a rut and sameness. Freshen up your day-to-day with Chestnut Bud.

Gemini: Madia Mental Magic for Twins

Curious Geminis are can overwork their brains by engaging in research and analysis to the point of overthinking. Preserve your intellectual power with a mental balancing tonic. Madia may be a great flower essence to try, as it's said to calm the waves of a wandering mind.

Cancer: Honeysuckle Health for Crabs

There are two sides to every coin, and that is so true here. Cancerians have a legendary love of history; so much so that they can start living there. Resist the pull of the past with Sweet Honeysuckle essence.

Leo: Borage for Brave Lions

Loving, giving, and so dramatic, Leos leave nothing behind as they live life full tilt. This can be emotionally exhausting and may also lead to many a heartbreak. When this happens, anyone, but especially Leos, will benefit from borage flower essence, which offers encouragement and can move you from sad and hurt to healing and openhearted.

Virgo: Pine Helps Perfectionists

Sticklers by nature, Virgoans work hard to be organized, on time, and have things just so. None of us are perfect, so that can be a set up for failure when you fail to meet your own extremely high standards, as it can lead to a swirl of negative self-talk. To get out of this cycle of negativity, Virgos can reconnect to self-compassion with pine essence.

Libra: Scleranthus Serenity

Our favorite Librans are often caught in a balancing act of weighing—and reweighing—their options before they make a decision. This can lead to vacillating in a cycle of indecision. To spur more decisive determination, try Scleranthus flower essence for more clear thinking and real balance.

Scorpio: Holly Is Holy

Scorpios have the height of intensity within them and are also tops in passions. This can lead to heartache, disappointment, upset and, even anger. Evergreen holly helps you feel the eternal love from the universe and brings balance to your life. If you feel like you are bumping up again endless frustration, tap into holly's holy life-giving energy.

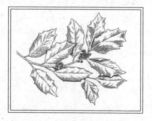

Sprig of holly

Sagittarius: Vervain Gives Vivacity

Sagittarians often feel like Energizer bunnies. While sharing your ideals with others fuels your spirit of *joie de vivre*, your ardent enthusiasm can sometimes have you setting overly optimistic goals. If you need support in balancing impassioned pursuits with a pragmatic perspective, try vervain flower essence.

Capricorn: Oak Prevents Overwhelm

Our loveable goats are unbelievably strong, but that can lead to never stopping (even when rest is really needed) and burnout. Capricorns also try to do everything on their own, drawing too much on their own can-do spirit, yet this can be a grueling path to getting to your goals and achievements. Oak is a marvelous flower essence helps with boundaries, energy preservation, and maintaining and not draining yourself while you get to the top of that mountain.

Aquarius: California Wild Rose

Water Bearers are the most unique of individuals. However, forging your own path and all that freethinking can create distance between you and others. You can become too detached from people, even your loved ones. You can also separate from staying grounded in practicality in your own life. When you feel gaps growing from disregarded aspects of your existence, turn to California wild rose, which will reenergize your sense of purpose and your ties to the important things in life.

Pisces: Pink Yarrow

While our favorite fish are deeply empathetic to the point of being psychic, their big issue can be boundaries. When you begin to feel other people's feelings too much, this causes emotional muddles, sadness, depression, anxiety, and ongoing overwhelm. Sensitivity and compassion are beautiful as long as you can draw and maintain clear boundaries between yourself and others. Pink Yarrow helps Pisces maintain mental clarity, good self-esteem, and healthy relationships.

Aloe: Skin-Soothing Solution

One of Mother Nature's most effective healers is aloe. When I lived in colder areas with frost and snow, I grew aloe in a wide pot with good drainage and placed it in the sunniest spot in the kitchen, where it thrived with very little water. I am truly fortunate to live where it never gets below freezing, so I have a towering aloe in the left garden corner that is growing to tree-like proportions. When anyone in the household gets a burn, a bug bite, a rash, a scratch, an itch, or a sunburn, I march back and grab a piece, slice parallel with its flat side, and apply the juice liberally. We use it as a medicine as well as a beauty application for facials, hair gel, and skin massage and feel so blessed that all this heavenly healing is utterly free of cost. Aloe propagates through baby plants sprouting off the sides; you can repot the "babies" into little clay containers and give them as gifts to your circle to share the healing energy as well as protection and luck

Sage Wisdom

Every kitchen gardener should grow an indoor pot of sage, if not a big patch in your garden. Sage is a must to have on hand for clearing energy. It also increases psychic potential. Whether your passion is growing an artful garden, throwing pots, cookery, or music, you can stay in better touch with your personal muse or guardian spirit with an aromatic sage wand. Head out to your garden or the sunny spot on the deck where your hardiest sage grows. Take three large and extra-long sticks of your favorite incense and bind strands of sage around the incense with purple thread. Tie it off, let it dry, and you have a sage wand. Before any creative endeavor, you can light this wand and wave it around your workspace, filling the area with inspiration. (Use a medium-size shell or bowl to catch any ashes or loose sage leaves as you cense your space.) Close your eyes and meditate upon the healing work you will begin.

Mint Refreshes Body and Mind

Another useful herb is mint, which comes from the Latin *menthe*, which literally means thought. Mint is so easily grown that a little bunch in the backyard can go on to become a scentful, attractive groundcover. It is also called the flower of eternal refreshment. Woven into a wreath, it bestows brilliance, artistic inspiration, and prophetic ability. As a tea, it accomplishes miracles of calming the stomach and the mind at the same time.

Comfrey for Comfort

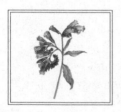

Comfrey is beloved by healers and is one of the best-known healing herbs of all times. It has even been referred to as "a one-herb pharmacy" for its inherent curative powers. Well-known to and widely used by the early Greeks and Romans, its very name, *symphytum*, from the Greek *symphyo,* means to "make grow together," referring to its traditional use of healing fractures. Comfrey relieves pain and inflammation, and comfrey salve will be a mainstay of your home first aid kit. Use it on cuts, scrapes, rashes, sunburn, and almost any skin irritation. Comfrey salve can also bring comfort to aching arthritic joints and sore muscles.

Emotional Rescue Remedy

Why does every day seem like it is a week long nowadays? Unplugging from cable news and constant social media feeds will help, as will this time-tested aromatherapy healing potion. This remedy is an excellent way to recharge and refresh after a hectic week. This tincture is most potent right after the sun sets, by the light of the moon.

In a small ceramic or glass bowl, gently mix together the following essential oils with a small amount of base carrier oil:

- ≫ 2 drops bergamot
- ≫ 4 drops carrier oil (apricot or sesame, ideally)
- ≫ 2 drops vanilla
- ≫ 1 drop amber
- ≫ 2 drops lavender

Take off your shoes so you can be more grounded. Walk outside, stand on your deck, or find a spot by an open window. Now, close your eyes, lift your head to the moon, and recite aloud:

> *Bright moon goddess, eternal and wise, give your strength to me now.*
>
> *As I breathe, you are alive in me for this night.*
>
> *Health to all, calm to me.*
>
> *So mote it be.*

Gently rub one drop of Calm Emotion Potion on each pulse point: on both wrists, behind your ear lobes, at the base of your neck, and behind your knees. As the oil surrounds you with its warm scent, you will be filled with a quiet strength.

Air Cleaners You Can Grow

Plants provide a haven, even in a small studio apartment. They are a great idea for at home as well as at work. Not only are they pretty to look at, they are improving the air you breathe. These air-purifying plants look great, produce oxygen, and can even absorb contaminants like formaldehyde and benzene, which are commonly off-gassed from furniture and mattresses. Here are the plants to purify the air in your home twenty-four-seven: bamboo, weeping figs, rubber tree, spider plant, peace lily, and snake plants. Houseplants do need their leaves dusted from time to time, so you can do this with a banana peel. The dust clings to the peel, and the leaves are nourished by the peel. Go bananas!

Sowing Seeds of Positive Change in Your Life

Nature is the ultimate creator. At a nearby gardening store or hardware store, get an assortment of seed packets to plant newness into your life. If your thumb is not the greenest, try nasturtiums, which are extremely hardy, grow quickly, and will spread to beautify any area. They reseed themselves, which is a lovely bonus. Light the following candles:

- ⋙ Green candle with a peridot or jade for creativity, prosperity, and growth

- ⋙ Orange candle with jasper or onyx for clear thinking and highest consciousness

- ⋙ Blue candle with turquoise or celestine for serenity, kindness and a happy heart

- ⋙ White candle with a quartz crystal or limestone for purification and safety

Put the seeds under the soil with your fingers and tamp them down gently with your fingers while meditating on your wish for positive changes. Water your new moon garden, and affirmative change will begin in your life that very day.

Garden Your Way to Gladness

For dispelling negative energy, plant heather, hawthorn, holly, hyacinth, hyssop, ivy, juniper, periwinkle, and nasturtiums.

For healing, plant sage, wood sorrel, carnation, onion, garlic, peppermint, and rosemary.

Both farming and working with plants are guided by the moon and should take place during the waxing moon in the signs of Cancer, Scorpio, Pisces, Capricorn, and Taurus, while weeding is ideally done during the waning moon.

Your Local Free Farmer's Market

If you are lucky enough to live nearby an untended meadow, you have a garden at your beck and call. Rocket, sorrel, nettles, dandelions, and purslane are there for the taking, along with the beautiful tall flowering weed Queen Anne's lace, the roots of which are tiny wild carrots. Foraging is good exercise as well as an exercise in economy, as these tasty weeds are free for the picking. All these greens are good for you, and purslane is a genuine superfood, one very high in omega-3 fatty acids. Foraging these wild wonderful weeds is a part of the centuries-old village tradition.

Magic by the Bushel

The very act of growing your own herbs will be healing, and, as you continue to practice herbalism, you will learn more and more of what works in your recipes and which herbs, teas, and plant-based potions and infusions cause you and your loved ones to flourish.

CHAPTER TWO

Grow Your Healing Garden: Herbs and Veggies

. . . .

I have lived in homes where my only gardening options were containers on a deck or planters on the front stoop. This taught me you can do a lot with seed packets, pots, and an open mind. When selecting space for your kitchen garden, you can plant it in something as simple as a set of containers; this can be planned as with any other garden space. If you are lucky to have a backyard or land, I suggest you begin the designing process by incorporating all the plants you know you want to use in your health and body care, your magical workings, and your cookery and always allow yourself to experiment. Trying new veggies or seeds that are new to you can be enormously rewarding. I agree with Londoner Alys Fowler, who is one of England's top gardeners. She says there is no earthly reason why roses and cabbages can't go side by side and that veggies can nicely nestle in among florals. Once you have tried a few such painterly plantings, you can give yourself a free hand in your creative approach.

Lawns are very high maintenance and unless constantly mowed and manicured, can greatly reduce your home's curb appeal. Besides wasting water and taking up a lot of time, grass in your yard doesn't offer you anything back for all the demands it places on your time and pocketbook. Grass lawns also tempt many lawn keepers to use chemicals which are bad for all of us, especially the birds and the bees. Get creative and go at least a little wild. My next-door neighbor turned over the soil on their whole front lawn, tilled it, and planted potatoes, beets, asparagus, and squash. They love going into the front yard and harvesting fresh veggies for their daily meals. The pumpkins and other squash actually have beautiful foliage, and the flowers are stunning and edible as well. Last year, one of their crops grew to "Giant Pumpkin" size and it became the talk of the neighborhood as we watched it grow and grow. Needless to say, they had the best jack-o-lantern on the block and some fantastic pies to boot. I am heartened to see the new gardening philosophy of growing veggies, roots stocks, herbs, and berries right beside the roses and lilies. It is gorgeous and supports the bee populations to whom we owe so much.

Gardening, even if it is only a hanging basket of cherry tomatoes and a windowsill filled with herb pots, is a way for us as human beings to live grounded in nature and connected to Mother Earth, who provides all. It will definitely add pleasure to your life and a sense of calm. When I feel stressed, I go out back and do some weeding. It is my therapy, and I can immediately see the profit of my labors. The bigger my compost pile grows with weeds, the happier I am. I intend the same for you. With your garden, you are quite literally growing a bounty of blessings.

The Art of the Kitchen Garden

What veggies do you love? What are your favorite salad greens? The first rule is to plant what you will actually eat and feel proud to serve to guests. Take your herbal journal and list your preferred herbs, greens, fruits, and vegetables including root vegetables. Now, strike out anything you can buy really cheaply—no sense in using valuable space to for something easily available at a lower price than the cost to grow it. Another caution, check out your soil type. Carrots need deep, rich soil to grow well. If your lot is shallow and sandy soil, cross carrots off your list and look to surface crops like potatoes and beets instead.

Gardening Is the Key to Happiness (and It's Easy!)

Here are the vegetables anyone can grow, from beginners to pros with their own greenhouses:

Lettuce, peas, onions, beets, potatoes, beans, and radishes.

Lettuce leaves for your salads are the easiest edible crop to grow. A few varieties will be ready to harvest in weeks! Choose a seed mix that will give you a variety of leaves for different tastes, colors, and textures. For best results, sow in stages so you don't get loads all at once. Sow a couple of lanes every few weeks throughout the summer to ensure a continuous supply.

Once you are a pro with lettuce, grow spinach and rocket (a.k.a. arugula) for your salad bowl.

Peas are a trouble-free crop that can handle cooler weather, so you can skip the step of starting the seedlings indoors. Simply sow the seeds in the ground from March onwards and watch them thrive. The plants will need support—put in stakes or chicken wire attached to posts and occasionally wind the stems around the supports as they grow. Harvest your fresh peas from June to August—the more you pick; the more will grow.

Onions are problem free and easy to propagate. After your seedlings sprout, thin seedlings to an inch apart, and then thin again in four weeks to six inches apart. Onions are a staple for cooking, so you and your family will be grateful once you have established an onion patch in your kitchen garden.

Potatoes and beets are a high return for your labor. To me, the best way to grow both is the world's laziest way to garden; I remember reading about it when I was ten in a book by Thalassa Crusoe, a pioneering organic gardener. I was fascinated that you could grow root vegetables without even needing to turn any soil. You can grow potatoes, yams, and so on under straw! Simply cut up mature potatoes that have "eyes" or the fleshy tubers sprouting out of the flesh of the potato, making sure each piece has an eye. This will give a new potato. After you "plant" or place the seed potatoes chunks on the ground, put loose straw over the pieces and between all the rows at least four to six inches deep. When the seed pieces start growing, your potato sprouts will emerge through the straw cover. How easy was that? Crusoe also said you could do the same under wet, shredded newspaper, but straw is more organic.

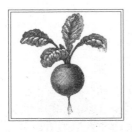

Radishes have enjoyed a new popularity thanks to Korean and Japanese cuisine. They add a fun pop of spicy, tangy flavor to soups, stews, tempura, salads, and all on their own. They can grow equally well in the ground in spring or in a pot. Radishes like a lot of sun and well-drained soil. They are also a crop you can grow in several crops per season. If you keep the soil moist, you'll have big beautiful radishes to brighten any dish.

Green beans are the opposite of the low-maintenance beets and potatoes as they will need staking or poles for support. However, an easier path to a great crop of green beans can be to grow them in a five-gallon container. After they have gotten four or five feet long, place a pole or stake carefully in the pot and allow the bean vines to wind around. Soon you'll have a pot of beans even grandma might recognize as a favorite vegetable for any occasion.

Invite Your Garden to Tea: How to Make Compost Tea

Compost tea is a marvelous way to feed your plants and give them extra nutrients in a wholly natural way that is free of chemicals. You want to feed your friends and family only the cleanest and pesticide-free produce, so start out organic and you will have a garden that produces healthy food. You will need a big bucket and the following to make compost tea:

- ⫸ 2 cups fresh, homemade compost dirt
- ⫸ 1 gallon of clean, filtered water

Add the water and the soil to a gallon bucket, and keep it in a place out of direct heat or cold. I use my outdoor shed, but a garage will also do nicely. Let your compost tea "brew" for a week, and give it a stir every other day. Watering cans are the perfect teapot for your garden. Strain out the dirt and pour the liquid into your watering can, where it will then be ready to serve up some serious nutrients to your garden.

An Herbalist's Green Thumb Rules

If you have children, get them involved so they will learn a love of gardening early.

Find a nursery you like and ask which is the best book for your zone and climate to read and understand what to plant where, so you'll have the best chance for success.

Always grow vegetables and fruits that you and your family love to eat.

Your kitchen garden should be a sunny, open spot that is easy for you to see and tend.

If possible, have an herb garden that is separate and easy to access for daily use when warm.

Check your soil type and use containers or raised beds if your soil is too poor or damp and swampy. Of course, a compost pile can fix your soil soon enough.

Preparation is everything, even with soil. Remove rocks and weeds; loosen the soil so it "breathes."

Develop your garden's soil by mixing in compost. Once the plants are established, serve them compost tea!

Patience is a virtue. Don't sow too early—wait until the soil is warmed up.

Harvesting Joy: Your Herb Garden

Basil is beloved because it's so delectable and versatile. It is easily grown in pots. Take care to remove the growing tip when the plants are six inches (fifteen cm) high for bushier growth. Plant out in the garden when the weather gets warmer. Basil prefers full sun and a sheltered spot.

Chives come from the onion family and have slim, pointed leaves. You should sow seeds directly in the ground in early spring, late March or April. Chives grow best in a sunny spot with rich soil, so keep the plants watered. Chives produce pretty, perfectly round flowers in either purple or pink. Gorgeous in the garden and palatable on the plate, the chive plant is a marvelous cooking herb and one that is truly easy to grow.

Coriander is a very versatile herb for the kitchen and grows well in the garden or in pots. Seeds can take weeks to germinate and the plants are fairly short-lived, so sow seeds every few weeks to get you through the season. Coriander is a bit fussy and can "bolt" when stressed, which means it produces flowers and seeds and not enough of the flavorful leaves. You need to make sure it is well watered and reap regularly before it goes to seed.

Mint is a marvel. It spreads beautifully once it has really taken root. If space is a concern, plant your mint in pots to contain the roots and stop it taking over. Keep it in full sun or partial shade and pinch out any flower buds to encourage more leaf growth.

Oregano loves a Mediterranean clime. Plant yours in warm, sunny spots with light soil. Oregano has pretty pink flowers and makes great ground cover at the front of borders. Don't allow this herb to get too tall; make sure to pinch it back, and you'll get more of this tasty treat to harvest.

Parsley is the gift that gives for two years. This herb can be slow to germinate; try soaking the seeds in water overnight before planting as this will speed it up. The best place to grow parsley is in rich, moist soil in full sun or partial shade.

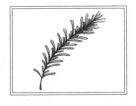

Rosemary is useful for so many culinary and healing teas and brews. Lucky for us, it grows vigorously. Rosemary can be trimmed in early summer to keep it in shape and stop it getting too woody. The scent is so wonderful in dishes and in bath salts, too!

Sage doesn't like wet ground, so plant it in a sunny spot with rich, well-drained soil. There are several sage varieties to choose from, including some with colored leaves. Harvest the leaves regularly to encourage more to grow. This versatile herb is a major culinary pleasure.

Thyme is a cousin of mint but grows much lower to the ground; it is one of the most fragrant of herbs and really adds flavor as a culinary seasoning. Plant this to remove melancholy from your home and garden. If your front yard and door get afternoon sun, plant wooly thyme and you'll come home after work to a perfume paradise that will immediately lend cheer and comfort.

All of these herbs will grow happily in containers on a patio, balcony, or even on the kitchen windowsill. Start an herb garden this year and you'll never look back.

Blissful Blend: Basil-Infused Oil

Infusions have regained popularity as a way of getting as much of the herb into oil as possible. This is a method of preparation that brings the flavors of one food, in this case, fresh herbs, to another, such as oil. Basil oil is unbelievably easy to make. You'll need:

- 2 ounces fresh basil
- ¾ cup virgin olive oil (or you can use safflower oil or canola)

Ideally, you will gather your fresh herbs in your own kitchen garden, but any farmers market or organic grocery will have green herbs. For the best and purest flavor, use fresh herbs at their peak. Rinse thoroughly in cold water. Gently pat dry with paper towels and give the basil a coarse chop. Place into a metal colander and dip into boiling water for ten seconds. Rinse in an ice water bath and drain well. Gently pat dry and add the basil to the oil. After three to five days in a cool dark place, the flavor will have infused into the oil, adding the fresh bright green note of the herbs. Use liberally on roasts, stir-frys, or salads, and drizzle on top of cooked vegetables and soups. Basil not only confers much palatability, but it also brings prosperity. Enjoy!

These herbs also make fantastic infused oils: rosemary. tarragon, parsley, chives, and cilantro.

The Herbalist's Astrological Almanac—Plant Healing Wisdom

Plants carry potent energy you can use to amplify your magical workings. Use the signs of the sun, moon, and stars to your advantage and, over time, you will come to know which ones are most effective for you. Make sure to use your own astrological chart in working with these herbs. Here is a guide to the astrological associations of plants you may grow in your kitchen garden or keep dried in your pantry:

- ⇜ **Aries**, ruled by Mars: carnation, cedar, clove, cumin, fennel, juniper, peppermint, and pine

- ⇜ **Taurus**, ruled by Venus: apple, daisy, lilac, magnolia, oak moss, orchid, plumeria, rose, thyme, tonka bean, vanilla, and violet

- ⇜ **Gemini**, ruled by Mercury: almond, bergamot, mint, clover, dill, lavender, lemongrass, lily, and parsley

- ⇜ **Cancer**, ruled by the moon: eucalyptus, gardenia, jasmine, lemon, lotus, rose, myrrh, and sandalwood

- ⇜ **Leo**, ruled by the Sun: acacia, cinnamon, heliotrope, nutmeg, orange, and rosemary

- ⇜ **Virgo**, ruled by Mercury: almond, cypress, bergamot, mint, mace, moss, thyme, and patchouli

- ⇜ **Libra**, ruled by Venus: catnip, marjoram, mugwort, spearmint, sweet pea, thyme, and vanilla

- ⇜ **Scorpio**, ruled by Pluto: allspice, basil, cumin, galangal, and ginger

◈ **Sagittarius**, ruled by Jupiter: anise, cedarwood, sassafras, star anise, and honeysuckle

◈ **Capricorn**, ruled by Saturn: lemon thyme, mimosa, vervain, and vetiver

◈ **Aquarius**, ruled by Uranus: gum, citron, cypress, lavender, spearmint, and pine

◈ **Pisces**, ruled by Neptune: clover, orris, neroli, sarsaparilla, and sweet pea

For the ingredients above not found in your kitchen or garden, try your local health food market, herbalist, or metaphysical store; for those that are really hard to find, consider looking at these types of mail-order outlets online.

Coziness by the Cup: Ambrosial Brews

Herbal tea conjures a very powerful alchemy because when you drink it, you take the magic inside. For an ambrosial brew with the power to calm any storm, add a sliver of ginger root and a pinch each of chamomile and peppermint to a cup of hot black tea. Before you drink, pray:

> *This day I pray for calm, for health,*
> *And the wisdom to see the beauty of each*
> *waking moment.*
> *Blessings abound.*

Herbal teas can also nourish the soul and heal the body:

Blueberry Leaf Tea

Reduces mood swings, evens glucose levels, and helps varicose veins.

Nettle

Raises the energy level, boosts the immune system, and is packed with iron and vitamins.

Fennel

Awakens and uplifts, freshens the breath, and aids colon health.

Echinacea

Supports an increased and consistent sense of well-being and prevents colds and flu.

Ginger Root

Calms and cheers while preventing nausea and aiding digestion and circulation.

Dandelion Root

Grounds and centers, provides many minerals and nutrients, and cleanses the liver of toxins.

CHAPTER THREE

Eating Healing Food: From Seed to Savory Meal

· ·

Centuries ago, healers were the wise women of the village, herbalists and midwives who could halt a fever with a poultice or hasten the setting of bones by concocting a medicinal tea. The lore of growing and gathering healing herbs has been passed down for hundreds of years. A learned herbal healer knows which phases of the moon are best for planting seeds, how to plan your garden by the stars, and how to create concoctions for health and harmony.

In the grand and hallowed tradition, I learned at the knee of my aunt Edith, a very wise woman who would take me for walks through the woods and show me the uses and meanings of every flower, weed, and tree. From her, I learned that lovely Queen Anne's lace is in fact wild carrot; that pokeberries make the finest blood-red inks; and which meadow greens and shade-loving mushrooms are safe for a noonday salad. I was in awe during our tromps through the woods, walking mile upon mile to map every acre and spy every specimen. Nature was our cathedral, our classroom, and our calendar. Every spring, we could mark April 1 by the blossoming of a solitary clump of delicate Dutchman's breeches amid a raft of rarest wildflowers. I thought Aunt Edith was teaching me about plants and trees, only to discover years later that she had shown me the sanctity of life and passed on to me a legacy I now treasure.

Herbal healing is "earth magic." These recipes that create both soundness of body and clarity of mind are eminently practical. They are a wonderful mix of gardening, herb lore, minding the moon and sky, and heeding ancient folk wisdom. In crafting herbal remedies for healing, you are using your magic in conjunction with the properties of the herbs—a powerful combination. It is a subtle process, growing more effective over tike through repeated practice.

Prior to modern medical science, it was believed that illness was a sign of evil spirits. A modern healer knows that most maladies come from myriad causes with such common roots as neglect, imbalance, stress, lack of sleep, and substance abuse, which includes eating the wrong types of foods. A good healer knows that prevention is always better than a cure and that self-care can greatly amplify the body's powerful self-healing properties. Your well-being is inextricably linked to the physical and spiritual health of the people around you, which in turn is connected to the planet at large. Thus, the healing process begins with you and spirals outward. The purifying positions and restorative herbal cures recounted in these pages provide a sacred road map to bring you in harmony with yourself and with the greater forces of nature. Many plants now thought of as weeds have great healing powers and magical properties. Most of the herbs and essential oils in this book have become quite commonplace. With the new plethora of aromatherapy products now available, most oil essences and scented candles can be bought commercially. For the more unusual ingredients, try your local health food market, herbalist or metaphysical store.

Healing Spices

Did you know your pantry is like a pharmacy? Thankfully, it is far cheaper. *Cumin* **is** loaded with phytochemicals, antioxidants, iron, copper, calcium, potassium, manganese, selenium, zinc, and magnesium and contains high amounts of B-complex nutrients. Cumin also helps with insomnia. *Cinnamon* is truly a power spice. Just half a teaspoon daily can dramatically reduce blood glucose levels in those with type 2 diabetes and lower cholesterol. *Cayenne* promotes circulation and boosts metabolism. *Clove* is an antifungal and abets toothaches. Nutrient-rich *parsley* is a detoxifying herb and acts as an anti-inflammatory and antispasmodic as well as helping conditions from colic to indigestion. Rub it on itchy skin for instant relief! *Sage* is very beneficial in treating gum and throat infections. Sage tea has helped ease depression and anxiety for generations. *Thyme* is a cure for a hangover and doubles as a remedy for colds and bronchitis. *Cilantro* is a good source of iron, magnesium, phytonutrients, and flavonoids and is also high in dietary fiber. Cilantro has been used for thousands of years as a digestive and helps to lower blood sugar when it is too high, possibly as a result of stimulating insulin secretion or enzyme production. *Ginger* stimulates circulation and is an excellent digestive as it aids in absorption of food and clears bloating due to indigestion. Immune champion *turmeric* boosts production of antioxidants and reduction of inflammation. Blue Zone centenarians credit their long, healthy lives to drinking turmeric root tea daily. Pack your pantry with these seasonings for optimal health and happiness.

I also had the great good fortune to have grown up in the countryside on a farm. Much of what I know I learned from my wise aunt: what herbs to gather in the wild and which foods to cook for love, money, luck, health, and in celebration of the high holidays. It is exciting to go to the garden, the grocery store, or the farmer's market and bring home the ingredients for positive life change. In addition to the secrets of magical cooking, I learned from this wise woman that the first task to undertake is to clean your kitchen and purify it. If anything needs repairing, fix it. Any utensils, pots, or pans that are banged up can also be donated (so long as you can afford to immediately purchase replacements). If your kitchen curtains look shabby to your eye, make or buy new ones. If there is a bag of rice or beans past its prime, compost away. You should both clean the cooking space in the practical sense as well as cleanse it in the magical sense. Prepare your kitchen to be used for the purpose of healing,

Healing in a Bowl: Ginger Carrot Soup

Ginger is an energetic herb, and it adds a bit of fire and spice to anything in which it is used, whether that is a healing cup of tea, a salad, a savory dish, or this special soup. Ginger root is a quickener and is renowned for how it can make magic happen faster. It is also medicinal and helps heals from colds, congestions, flus, and fever. Combine ginger with carrots, which are wonderfully grounding and bring what is hidden to light, and you have a simple soup that can ground and center you, heal you, and make you more psychic—all at a faster pace. And as if that wasn't enough, it is beautiful to smell and to see and is pleasing to the senses in all ways. This is what you need for this bowlful of soothing soup:

- ⟫ 1 pound of carrots, cleaned and sliced; set aside the carrot greens
- ⟫ 1 tablespoon fresh ginger, chopped
- ⟫ 1 large clove garlic, peeled and crushed
- ⟫ ¼ teaspoon crushed red pepper, extra for garnish
- ⟫ ½ teaspoon salt
- ⟫ 4 cups fresh water
- ⟫ 1 lemon

Put all the carrots except for one in a big pot and cover with water; simmer on medium heat and add in the ginger, garlic, pepper, and salt after the first five minutes. Place the last carrot on your altar. After twenty to twenty-five minutes, the carrots should be tender. Transfer everything to a blender and blend until smooth. At the very end, add in several squeezes of lemon juice.

Give a stir and pour into bowls or mugs while nice and warm. Use a few leaves from the carrot tops and a tiny sprinkling of red pepper as garnish.

Grow Your Own Vitamins

This easy-to-grow delight provides several nutrients essential to maintaining overall health, including manganese and vitamin C, and it makes for vibrant skin. Here is a short and sweet recipe for a refreshingly cold soup to share with loved ones on a hot day.

Cool as a Cucumber Mint Soup

- ≫ 3 large peeled cucumbers
- ≫ Half cup fresh mint leaves
- ≫ 1 teaspoon kosher salt
- ≫ 3 tablespoons olive oil

Put the ingredients in the blender and puree. This gorgeous green potage makes four cups, enough for two servings for a hungry couple. The only accompaniment you need is crispy herb crackers, an icy beverage and each other.

Healing Moon Herb Soup

After the September Equinox signals the change of seasons to fall, you should start making pots of this seasonal meal, which is a guaranteed crowd pleaser. This autumnal soup is just as pleasing to the cook as it can be a quick supper, leftovers for lunch, and easily frozen for meals on the go. It is simple and simply delicious. On the eve of the first full moon of fall, gather the ingredients and prepare this nourishing lunar tonic. Refrigerate overnight, and the flavors will "marry" together to intensify and become an even more savory supper to serve to loved ones on a Harvest Moon night.

- 1 butternut squash, peeled, seeded, and shredded
- 3 large, thinly sliced leeks
- 2 cloves fresh garlic
- 8 cups of water
- ⅓ cup of virgin olive oil
- ¼ cup sage, finely ground
- 4 large potatoes cut into small, spoon-size chunks; they can be yams, purple Peruvian potatoes, Idaho spuds, red potatoes—cook's choice!
- ¼ cup fresh chives diced and chopped finely
- ¼ teaspoon celery salt
- Salt and pepper to your taste
- 1 carrot sliced thin into golden moons

In a large iron skillet (preferably one well-seasoned by use in your kitchen), fry the leeks in the olive oil until they become soft and translucent. Add in the chopped garlic until it is also soft and is wafting a wonderful scent into your kitchen. Transfer to a soup pot, oil and all, and add the water, heating to a boil. Add all the remaining veggies, the garlic, and the herbs, then turn the heat down to a simmer for forty-five minutes. Test the taters to see if they are soft enough by mashing a couple with a wooden spoon. If they are still a bit hard, simmer for another five minutes. Turn the heat down to very low and then season with salt and pepper to taste. Add the celery salt as the last element of the year's abundance.

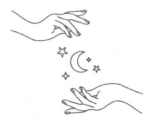

Lunar Almanac: Twelve Months of Full Moons

Many of our full moon names come from medieval books of hours and from Native American tribal traditions. Here is a list of rare names from these two branches of tradition that you may want to use in your lunar rituals.

January: Old Moon, Chaste Moon; this fierce Wolf Moon is the time to recognize your strength of spirit.

February: Hunger Moon; the cool Snow Moon is for personal vision and intention-setting.

March: Crust Moon, Sugar Moon; the gentle Sap Moon heralds the end of winter and nature's rebirth.

April: Sprouting Grass Moon, Egg Moon, Fish Moon; spring's sweet Pink Moon celebrates health and full life force.

May: Milk Moon, Corn Planting Moon, Dyad Moon; the Flower Moon provides inspiration with the bloom of beauty.

June: Horn Moon, Rose Moon; the Strawberry Moon heralds the Summer Solstice and the sustaining power of the sun.

July: Buck Moon, Hay Moon; this Thunder Moon showers us with rain and cleansing storms.

August: Barley Moon, Wort Moon, Sturgeon Moon; summer gifts us with the Red Moon, the time for passion and lust for life.

September: Green Corn Moon, Wine Moon; fall's Harvest Moon is the time to be grateful and reap what we have sown.

October: Dying Grass Moon, Travel Moon, Blood Moon, Moon of Changing Seasons; the Hunter's moon is when we plan and store for winter ahead.

November: Frost Moon, Snow Moon; this Beaver Moon is the time to call upon our true wild nature.

December: Cold Moon, Oak Moon; this is the longest night of the shortest day and is the time to gather the tribe around the fire and share stories of the good life together.

WeMoon Sweet Potato Cakes

Hearty and oh-so-healthy, these pancakes make for a marvelous full moon meal. Sweet potatoes are truly beneficial to women's health and contain estrogen; these tubers are good for you inside and out, as they also give your skin a nice boost. But their main magic for folks of all ages and genders is that they are a grounding tonic. Anytime you feel spacey, out of sorts, or distracted, this food will serve you well, even if you just bake and eat a sweet potato. For this savory sweet, you will need:

- ⟫ 2 large semi-baked sweet potatoes, peeled and grated
- ⟫ 1 large carrot, grated
- ⟫ 2 large semi-baked russet potatoes, peeled and grated
- ⟫ 3 eggs
- ⟫ ½ cup olive oil
- ⟫ 1 cup of yogurt (organic will taste best)
- ⟫ Chives, sage, and rosemary

Mix the grated potatoes and carrot in a large bowl. Beat the eggs, then add to the veggie mixture and mix thoroughly. Grind the rosemary and sage to a very fine powder in your mortar and pestle and add in a tablespoon of the herbs to the mixture; salt and pepper to taste. Shape into round balls, enough for eight mooncakes. Warm the oil slowly until it is nice and hot. Place the balls in the oil and flatten into rounds with a spatula. Cook through until they are golden and beginning to crisp on both sides. Plate up and top with organic yogurt, garnishing with chives. If you are feeling decadent, dollop on some sour cream and enjoy with a circle of friends under the sheen of a bright and holy moon.

Sara's Superfood Smoothie

A friend of mine came up with this delicious and nutritious smoothie so her daughter could get "everything" at once. Sara loves it, and so do we!

- 1 banana
- ½ cup strawberries, sliced
- 4 tablespoons plain yogurt
- 1 tablespoon liquid chlorophyll
- 1 tablespoon hemp oil
- ½ cup orange juice
- 2 tablespoons goji berries, presoaked (optional)
- 1 packet Emergen-C, or another vitamin C powder

If you are using goji berries, soak them for two hours before you make the smoothie.

Blend ingredients until smooth. Add a little more orange juice or water if the consistency is too thick for your taste.

Winter Is Coming Nut Roast

Nuts are some of the best food we humans can eat, packed as they are with positive proteins, beneficial oils, and delicious flavor. This nearly effortless nut roastie is a great snack either for movie night at home or party time, and it makes a savory appetizer for special meals. Here is what you need:

- 10 ounces mixed nuts
- 8 ounces day-old bread
- 1 medium-sized white onion, chopped
- 1½ cups vegetable stock
- Soy or tamari sauce
- 2 ounces unsalted butter
- 1 teaspoon dried sage

Preheat your oven to 350 degrees and start sautéing the onions in the butter until they soften. Mix the nuts together with the bread in a food processor or stir vigorously until blended well, then transfer to a large bowl. Heat the stock to a boil and pour into the mixture in the bowl. Stir in the onions. Season as you see fit with salt, pepper, and sage. Pour in a tablespoon of the soy or tamari sauce to add zing to your roast and give one last stir. Spoon the roastie mix into a greased baking dish and bake for a half hour. Notice as your kitchen fills with a fantastic aroma. Heating the nuts brings out more of their natural oils and intensifies the flavor. Like herbs and flowers, nuts have magical properties which are mainly to increase love and feelings of conviviality and peace. When you serve this roastie, you are quite literally sharing the love.

Graceful Connection

Before you enjoy this friendly repast together, hold hands and recite this grace:

> *Sister, brother, tribe of the soul, ones who care.*
>
> *Merry may we meet again to share.*
>
> *Breaking bread and quaffing mead*
>
> *We draw closer in word and deed.*
>
> *Blessing of love to all!*

Farmer's Favorite Nettle Soup: Medieval Superfood for Modern Times

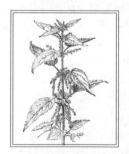

Nettles are a farmer's favorite due to all their usefulness as a healing plant bringing good cheer and for their usefulness in breaking hexes. They are also a green that can be used as you might use kale or watercress. They were regarded and used as a "superfood" by wise women for centuries and are so packed with vitamin A and iron, and they also have a high protein count. They are best harvested when they are young in the springtime. Nevertheless, they are an excellent element in cookery year 'round and have a surprisingly delicate flavor. They are another generous genus, since they sprout up and reseed themselves as true gifts from Mother Earth. Try this old-time recipe and you will be soon be out hunting nettles in the wild so you can enjoy this medieval meal at all times.

- ⇛ 2 cups rinsed nettles
- ⇛ 1 cup black-eyed peas, cleaned and soaked overnight
- ⇛ 3 cups vegetable stock
- ⇛ 2 garlic cloves, chopped
- ⇛ 2 cups yellow onions, chopped
- ⇛ ¼ cup olive oil
- ⇛ 1 teaspoon celery salt, salt and pepper to taste

Start cooking the presoaked black-eyed peas in a large pan with just enough water to cover them. Once they have boiled, keep them on a high simmer. Keep an eye on them while you sauté the onions and garlic to transparency in the olive oil in a skillet. Add water to the peas as needed and continue simmering them for thirty-five minutes or until the legumes have softened; then add the veggie stock or yeasty water.

Add the softened garlic and onions to the bean pot and simmer on low for twenty-five minutes. Add the nettles to the big pot and cook for a half hour. Season to taste and then share this nurturing soup. Make sure to give thanks to the guardian spirits of the earth for this gift of great greens.

Bounty of Basil: Perfect Pesto

This recipe is simply scrumptious and a bargain to boot. Gather a nice big bunch of basil leaves, two cups total, from your kitchen garden or greengrocer. Give the leaves a good cold rinse and place them on a clean tea towel to air-dry. You will also need the following:

- 1 fresh lemon
- 3 peeled garlic cloves
- ½ cup parmesan cheese
- ½ cup pine nuts
- Sea salt

Place the pine nuts and the garlic on a baking sheet in the oven at 375 degrees for five to ten minutes or until the pine nuts begin to turn slightly golden. Do NOT wait until they turn brown, though. Then take everything and put it into a blender or food processor. Before you put the lid in place, cut the lemon in half and squeeze out a nice dollop of fresh juice into the mix and grind in a healthy dash of sea salt. Blend away until you have a lovely green pesto sauce you can put on anything. Perfect pesto in ten minutes flat! Based on the benefits of this herb, it might be the perfect dish to serve up after an emotionally hard week as it is a bringer of peace. Also good for date night or when you need to brew up good money mojo! Boil up a pot of pasta while you are concocting the blissful basil blend, and you will have a sumptuous weeknight supper for the family on the table so quickly, they will be sure you are using witchcraft!

Hillbilly Health Food: Ramps!

As a West Virginian, I am very familiar with ramps and find it highly amusing that they are very on trend these days. An old-fashioned food that is now wildly fashionable, ramps were formerly the domain of hill folk and farm women. Even the chicest of city chefs have gone wild for ramps, which are akin to leeks and can be substituted for them in recipes. Ramps are more powerfully pungent than domesticated bulbs. The beauty of this recipe is that rice and ramps take only twenty minutes to cook. As winter thaws into spring, bulbs are the first to do the work of bringing forth the new season. This change-of-seasons dish combines risotto-style rice with a harbinger of spring to delightful effect. The old wives and village healers who were the first to explore ramps believed this healing green can prevent colds and flus.

- ➤ ½ cup sliced ramp bulbs
- ➤ 1½ cups long grain rice
- ➤ 3 tablespoons unsalted butter
- ➤ 3 cups unsalted organic chicken stock
- ➤ 1 teaspoon cayenne pepper
- ➤ ½ cup finely minced ramp greens

In a heavy saucepan, melt the butter over moderate heat. Toss in the sliced ramp bulbs and cook between three and five minutes until they soften, stirring gently. Add the rice to the pan and stir well to mix the rice, butter, and ramp bulbs well and get the rice sticky with the butter. After two minutes, add the chicken stock, salt, and cayenne pepper and stir thoroughly. Bring to a boil, then stir three times counterclockwise, turn the heat down low, and let simmer for twenty minutes. At that point, all the liquid should have been absorbed by the rice. Turn the heat off and stir half of the minced ramp greens into the rice. Pour the ramped-up rice into a serving bowl and sprinkle the rest of the minced greens on the top as a garnish.

Before you and your guests begin, stop and breathe in the aroma of the healing savory greens. This is also an occasion to share stories of the wise women and elders in your life and honor all they passed down.

New Potatoes 'n Parsley

Parsley has somehow become just a garnish, but it is actually the perfect party herbage as it is ruled by both Mercury and Venus and brings eloquence and extra charm. Bonus: it prevents drunkenness and is a proven breath freshener. Potatoes are centering and connote the prosperity principle of stability. New potatoes, especially those grown by your own hand, are optimal, but russet potatoes are fine here, too. This salad should not wait for picnics and parties, it is marvelous for any meal and quite economical, too. All you need is this:

- 6 large scrubbed-clean potatoes, boiled and cubed (with the skin left on for more nutrients)

- 1 large red onion, chopped finely

- Parsley and chives, a nice fresh bunch from the garden

- ¼ cup mustard
- 1 cup olive oil
- 2 tablespoons apple cider vinegar
- 1 tablespoon sugar
- 1 lemon

While the potatoes are cooling, place them in a large bowl and add in the onion. Whisk the lemon, vinegar, mustard, and sugar and then pour in the olive oil bit by bit. Pour most of the herbs and dressing into the still-warm potatoes and stir until the dressing is completely mixed in. Season to taste and top with the leftover herbs. This dish is a lovely tasting reminder of how the earth sustains us all.

Gardener's Choice Goddess Greens

This dish should be the gardener's choice with a big bunch of gorgeous greens:

- Kale or chard (with a suggested side of nettle)
- 2 small garlic cloves
- ¼ cup apple cider vinegar
- Red pepper flakes
- Garlic salt
- Olive oil

Wash the greens thoroughly, chop, and set aside. Peel and mash the garlic cloves. Heat the olive oil in a skillet and fry up the garlic and the pepper flakes. Add in the chopped greens and stir well. Cover the pan and lower the heat, giving it a stir every few minutes. When the greens have softened to your liking, add in a tablespoon of the apple cider vinegar and a big dash of the garlic salt. Stir vigorously three times counterclockwise and pray to the great kitchen goddess who provides us with everything we have. Remove from the heat. Lift the lid and add a half teaspoon of red pepper flakes. Serve this goddess-blessed dish of greens to people who claim to not like veggies or greens and you will delight and surprise quite a few. Be prepared to be asked for the recipe repeatedly. Every time you share the dish (or the recipe) you'll be sharing the gifts of the goddess directly.

Magical Mushroom Veggie Quiche

This dish can be either a main course served with a leafy green salad or a yummy hot breakfast or brunch with a side of fruit. Make two, and your weekend options are deliciously open. You can also include greens such as nettles, spinach, or chives to add more color and nutrients to your meal.

Gather the following ingredients:

- ⫸ 5 eggs
- ⫸ ½ cup milk

- ➤ 3 ounces cheese, grated (cook's choice of cheddar, Swiss, or another family favorite)

- ➤ ½ cup washed and sliced button or cremini mushrooms

- ➤ ½ cup of chopped greens

- ➤ A premade pastry or quiche shell in a greased pie pan (can be store-bought or handmade, depending on how much time you have)

Preheat your oven to 375 degrees. Whisk the eggs and milk together and season with salt and pepper. Fold in the grated cheese and stir in the mushrooms. Pour the mixture into the pastry shell and pop into the oven for thirty-five minutes. When the top is turning a nice golden brown, remove the quiche from the oven and let it cool. Top with sprigs of aromatic fresh rosemary from your kitchen garden.

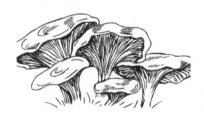

Mushrooms: An Anti-Cancer Food to Add to Your Meals

But just what is so magical about mushrooms? One cup of cremini mushrooms provides either a good, very good, or excellent source of fifteen different vitamins, minerals, and antioxidant phytonutrients. They have even been reported to be an anti-cancer food and aid in the reduction of high cholesterol. Some, like the shiitake mushrooms beloved of Japanese cuisine, even boost the immune system! Mighty magical indeed!

Savory Shepherd's Pie

This recipe is an old-school comfort food at its finest and is very filling and festive. Many of us are working mothers with very busy schedules, so it's good to make a double recipe of this family favorite. Make one to serve piping hot out of the oven, and freeze the second for an after-school and post-work reheated repast. You will need the following ingredients for one pie:

- 1 yellow onion, chopped
- ½ cup carrots, sliced
- 1 cup button mushrooms, sliced
- 1 cup cherry tomatoes (or tomato sauce)
- 4 to 5 potatoes, boiled (or for a keto/low carb alternative, use an equal weight of young turnips, which are quite tasty mashed)
- ½ cup milk
- 2 tablespoons sunflower or olive oil
- ½ cup grated Cheddar cheese
- 2 cups sautéed ground beef (or substitute soy protein for a meat-free option, or ground turkey for a lower fat meat)
- ⅓ stick unsalted butter (preferably organic for best taste)

❧   seasoning herbs (cook's choice; see below)

Preheat the oven to 375 degrees.

Mash the potatoes with unsalted organic butter, adding a splash of milk until you have the desired consistency. As you mash the potatoes, make sure you can get peaks so the pie will be impressively landscaped! Slowly heat the olive oil in a sauté pan and cook the onions until they soften, then fold in and cook your meat or veggie protein. Lastly, add in the carrots, mushrooms, and tomato and cook through. Season with salt and pepper to taste and add in your favorite herbs—parsley, sage, rosemary, or whatever your heart desires. Transfer to an oiled pie dish and spread evenly. Sprinkle the grated cheese on the filling. Lastly, spread the mashed potatoes on top, creating peaks and valleys. Dust a sprinkling of parsley and chives onto the potatoes and pop it into the preheated oven for fifteen minutes. Once the tater topping begins to turn a lovely golden brown on top, remove from the oven. Serve this hearty homemade savory pie in bowls alongside a crisp salad of homegrown greens and allow its coziness to melt all mundane matters away. Good for any day of the week and impressive enough to bake for high holidays.

Kombucha Tea

Some people love the taste of kombucha tea; others don't relish it at all. It has been credited with miraculous properties and is a probiotic, making it very curative for digestive issues. Kombucha also comes recommended for acne, constipation, arthritis, depression, and fatigue, and is hailed as a protection against cancer. I regard it as a tasty tonic, and my family drinks it daily. My nephews were the first of my kin to taste kombucha, and they loved its fizziness and flavor. This healthful drink is easy to make so long as you have a "ferment" (which some people call a "mushroom" because of the way it looks). To procure your ferment, try to find somebody who brews kombucha already. They should have plenty of ferments to share, as every batch of tea grows an extra ferment on top of the original. Before brewing your kombucha, you will need:

- ⤜ a large wide-necked glass jar, a cloth or paper towel to cover the jar, and a rubber band to secure the covering cloth or paper towel

- ⤜ 7 tea bags, either black or green (preferably organic)

- ⤜ 1 cup sugar

- ⤜ 2 quarts water

- ⤜ kombucha ferment

Boil the water and add it to the tea bags in the jar. Let it steep for twenty minutes.

Remove the tea bags and add the sugar, stirring to dissolve.

When the tea has cooled, add the kombucha ferment with some of the liquor that it came in, which should come out to roughly 10 percent of the total tea in your jar.

Cover the jar with the cloth or paper towel, securing your cover with the rubber band. The lid will serve to keep dust and flies out while still allowing the tea to breathe. Let the jar sit in one place (as moving can disturb the fermentation process), out of the direct sunlight and at room temperature.

The fermentation process will take seven to twelve days, depending on the temperature in the room. Your batch of kombucha will ferment more quickly if the room is warm. You have to check to see when it is ready, and you'll be able to tell by the taste. When fermented, the tea can be decanted into glass bottles with screw lids and kept in the fridge. Remember to keep a little of the kombucha tea to add to the next batch with your ferment.

CHAPTER FOUR

DIY Herbal Salves, Lotions, Potions, and Skin Soothers

Taking good care of your skin is truly good common sense. Staying hydrated by drinking enough water and light herbal teas is a good start, as is moisturizing with natural and organic lotions and salves, Gentle abrasives in the form of body scrubs are an excellent way to stimulate your skin, the largest organ of the human body. Massaging yourself with these is also good for the lymphatic system. It is extremely affordable and oh so easy to use what you already have on hand, such as brown sugar, baking soda, or coffee grounds, along with binding substances which keep the abrasives sticking together while you scrub. Binding substances can be oils such as almond oil, coconut oil, olive oil, or my personal favorite, sesame oil. You can use honey, too, if you don't mind a bit of stickiness. Let your imagination run wild with extras such as fragrance or appearance enhancers—spices, essential oils, or even flower petals.

Remedies at the Ready: Your Herbal Medicine Cabinet

I've found that my remedy box has grown into a cupboard over the years. I tend to study and read up on a condition and seek out the most effective and reliably recommended remedy to treat it. Most herbs, tinctures, and essential oils have more than one therapeutic use, and my knowledge has grown as a result of having some of these herbs in my cupboard. Often, the range of uses is wide; for example, lavender oil is indicated for skin conditions, respiratory and circulatory problems, nervous tension and exhaustion, coughs and colds, muscle aches, and menstrual cramps, as well as cuts. I stanched a deep cut on my toe with lavender oil recently, a new use for me, and it worked great. It's a natural disinfectant, too! I would estimate that this cure cost me about a dime as opposed to a two-thousand-dollar trip to a crowded emergency room, with exposure to myriad viruses. It was peace of mind for pennies.

I keep a well-stocked first aid kit. Instead of expensive over-the-counter products, we use hydrogen peroxide, witch hazel, calamine lotion, aloe vera gel, and both arnica cream and calendula cream. We are ready for (almost) anything!

Creams and ointments are often expensive to buy but can be made easily at home. Here is an easy recipe to make your own curative cream.

Make Your Own Topical Ointment

- one stainless steel saucepan, bowl, whisk, and cooking thermometer
- small clean jars or cans to store your ointment in
- 1 tablespoon (15 grams) beeswax
- 5 tablespoons (80 milliliters) organic vegetable oil (sunflower oil is effective and affordable; jojoba oil and avocado oil are nice, but pricey)
- Arnica tincture; add 30 drops of arnica tincture to make an arnica cream. OR Calendula tincture; add 30 drops of calendula tincture and 10 drops of lavender oil to make calendula cream

(Note that arnica, calendula, and lavender can all be harmoniously combined in whatever proportions you prefer.)

Melt the beeswax and vegetable oil in a double boiler (or in a bowl over a saucepan in a pinch). When the beeswax is fully melted, remove the pan from the heat. Whisk the ointment until it has cooled to around 100 degrees, then stir in the tincture you are using.

Label and store in clean, sealable, lidded jars or cans. Your homemade creams will last longest if you keep them refrigerated, especially when the weather is warm.

Sacred Self-Care Spa Scrubs

Here are some simple scrubs for you to try. Keep some sealable glass jars with lids handy so you can store them for up to two months. Be sure and rinse the tub and sink thoroughly after use to avoid stains or stickiness. Add pretty labels, and you'll have pretty and practical gifts for your gal pals!

Lemon Up

- ½ cup of white sugar
- 2 tablespoons lemon juice and 1 teaspoon of lemon rind zest
- 1 tablespoon olive oil

CocoColada Sugar Scrub

- 1 cup brown sugar
- 3 tablespoons melted coconut oil
- A teaspoon each of cinnamon and ground cloves

Morning Cup Coffee Scrub

- ½ cup coffee grounds
- ½ cup fine sea salt
- 1 to 2 tablespoons almond oil

Shea Soother:
Light as Air Lotion

Here is a real treat: a light creamy body lotion that glides on and does not feel heavy. Best of all? The delectable scents of almond and grapefruit. Anyone on your gift list will delight in this, as will your household. A mixer is ideal, otherwise use a hand whisk and wooden spoon, a lidded jar, and the following ingredients:

- ½ cup room temperature virgin coconut oil
- 2 tablespoons room temperature raw shea butter
- 2 cups almond oil
- 2 tablespoons red grapefruit zest
- 2 teaspoons tapioca flour

Place the shea butter, coconut oil, almond oil, and red grapefruit zest in the bowl of a mixer fitted with the whisk attachment. Mix on medium for half a minute. Now, turn to high and whip the lotion for about four minutes, until it is light and fluffy. Scrape the sides of the bowl as needed. Add in the tapioca flour and mix for one more minute. Transfer to a jar with a lid and store at room temperature for up to a month.

Once known as "the forbidden fruit of Barbados," grapefruit awakens the mind and body and speaks to the soul. Like many other citrus fruits, it is cheering and renowned for what it does for the skin, even reducing cellulite. Almond is beloved for bringing luck in love and is prized as an erotic massage oil. Coconut protects and purifies and enhances confidence. Coconut brings forth your real allure and beauty, so use it carefully!

Bless Your Body Meditation

Whenever you have made a batch of salts, scrubs, or magic potions, whether for your own use or as a gift, you should stop and count your health blessings with this mindfulness practice.

Sit in a comfortable position with your bottle of potions placed in a bowl or dish in front of you. Think about the blessings in your life and what gifts your particular item offers; visualize your skin and hair gleaming with vitality. Picture your loved ones wearing a big smile as they use your handmade remedies. What are you grateful for at this moment? There is a powerful magic in recognizing all that you possess and in having an attitude of gratitude. Breathe steadily and deeply, inhaling and exhaling slowly for twenty minutes. As you meditate, send the positive energy into the bowl containing your personal potions. Now, the blessings are there any time you or a loved one may need them.

Mother Nature's Beauty Secrets

The best beauty secrets are often hidden amongst Mother Nature's flora and fauna. Forget spending a fortune on overpriced creams, lotions, masks, and salves, go out to your kitchen garden or check your pantry for organic remedies and common beauty solutions. Here are some of the best recipes and natural ingredients to begin a journey toward a healthy and nontoxic beauty regime.

Very Vanilla Sugar Scrub

Sugar scrubs exfoliate the skin while helping it stay nourished with moisture. This recipe could not be simpler yet is a delightfully decadent DIY scrub in the tub.

All you need are four simple ingredients:

- ⋙ ¼ cup brown sugar
- ⋙ ¼ cup white sugar
- ⋙ ¼ cup organic olive oil
- ⋙ 6 to 8 drops Vanilla essential oil

Grab a small bowl and measure out equal parts white sugar and brown sugar. Start with ¼ cup of each type of sugar. Mix the sugars together thoroughly using a wooden spoon. Now, add in the olive oil—the amount used depends on your taste. Do use enough oil, though, to coat the sugar well and create a pliable texture. Lastly, add in a few drops of vanilla; I go with at least six drops. You can also try variations on the recipe with all brown sugar and various other essential oils. My absolute favorite is equal parts vanilla oil and amber oil, which I call "vamber." It is great to get ready for a date night out on the town. You will look and feel like the goddess of love herself.

Earthly Pleasure Sensual Scrub

Sandalwood, amber, and vetiver are all rich, earthy scents that combine well together.

- ⋙ 5 drops sandalwood essential oil
- ⋙ 5 drops amber essential oil
- ⋙ 2 drops vetiver essential oil
- ⋙ ½ cup Epsom salts
- ⋙ ½ cup baking soda

Combine the essential oils with the Epsom salts and stir in the baking soda. Mix well, and the mixture will become a richly scented paste. You can use it a couple of different ways; one is to slather it onto yourself and shower off with a loofah and thick washcloth. But my favorite way to soak up this earthly pleasure fully is to roll it into a ball after you mix it, then place the ball under the faucet as you are running a hot bath. The entire room will smell like paradise. Soak it all in, lie back, and enjoy the experience fully.

If you want to store some of this scrub for the future or give it as a thoughtful gift, you can store it in a lidded plastic one-cup container, or roll the mix into bath bomb balls and let the balls dry on wax paper or paper towels. This recipe can make three palm size bath bombs. Note: you will be asked for more!

No More Itchy, Dry Skin: Porridge Potion

Naturally calming oatmeal is one of the best solutions for irritated and itchy skin. Add a cup of well-ground oats tied up in a muslin bag to your bath to help soothe the pain and discomfort of sunburned skin. It is also good for rashes and helps get your skin back to a smooth and healthy condition.

Oatmeal Chamomile Mask

Two things you doubtless love to taste in the morning can also be an important part of your beauty regime, chamomile tea and warm oatmeal. Here's what you need to make the mask:

- ½ cup old-fashioned oats, ideally steel-cut, crushed into finer bits using a ricer
- 1 cup chamomile tea, steeped covered for a half hour
- 2 tablespoons brown sugar
- 1 teaspoon baking soda
- 1 tablespoon honey

Take a half cup of the brewed chamomile tea and add with the honey, baking soda, and oats in a small bowl. Now add 2 more tablespoons of tea and mix to create an oat paste. Set it aside for five minutes. If the mixture is too dry, you can get the desired texture by adding a bit more tea. Add the sugar and mix well. Apply the mask to your face after you have cleaned your skin and while it is still a bit damp. Allow it to dry on your face for ten minutes. Rinse the paste off your face well, then massage your skin gently with a natural moisturizer. Your skin will be miraculously smooth!

Orgasmic Oil

I use this potion as a combination body care oil and mystical massage oil. You will need:

- ➤➤➤ 1 cup of sesame oil (you can cheat and get the sesame-scented oil from the pharmacy or grocery store, which works just as well in a pinch)
- ➤➤➤ Clove, cinnamon, and ginger (powdered)
- ➤➤➤ Bergamot, amber, and jasmine essential oils
- ➤➤➤ Amber-colored jar
- ➤➤➤ Magnetite

Take the sesame oil and add a pinch of each of the spices. Then add a drop of citrusy bergamot and a teaspoon each of the amber and jasmine oils.

Stir gently and then place in an amber-colored jar with a stopper. Place the jar beside a piece of magnetite, also known as lodestone, which draws people to you. Let it sit for a full week, and then use it to bring great happiness into your life.

Yummy Spa Scrubs

Luxe Locks DIY Shampoo

for medium to oily hair only

- ➳ 1 cup warm water
- ➳ 1 tablespoon baking soda

Take a large bowl and pour the water in. Fold in the baking soda and stir well until it has dissolved. Now, pour it over your wet hair while in the bath or shower. Massage the mixture into your hair, paying special attention to the scalp. If you tend to have oily hair, concentrate your efforts around the hairline and at the crown of the head. If you have long hair, you can double up on the amounts. Rinse thoroughly.

Orchard Fresh Hair Conditioner

The goddess of orchards is Pomona, who is a protector of nature associated with love and beauty. You will be protecting your lovely locks by creating this simple yet effective DIY conditioner.

- ➳ 1 cup warm water
- ➳ 2 tablespoons apple cider vinegar

Mix both ingredients in a bowl and pour over freshly shampooed hair. Gently massage into your hair and scalp and leave for a few moments before rinsing. It's remarkable how well these two components work to clean and condition your hair. You save a mind-boggling amount of money, and your hair and your home will be healthier. After a couple of months of DIY hair love, your hair will be shockingly shiny. Place an apple on your altar, and offer your thanks to the goddess Pomona for her generosity and guardianship of fruit orchards around the world.

Witch Hazel Wisdom

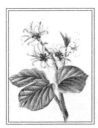 Witch hazel is an excellent and inexpensive astringent and antiseptic to always keep on hand. Topical uses for witch hazel include cleaning cuts, reducing skin inflammations and abrasions, sunburns, insect bites, bruising, poison oak and ivy, diaper rash, eczema, varicose veins, and hemorrhoids.

Preparations of witch hazel from the pharmacy generally contain isopropyl alcohol, so make sure you only use it externally, as it is poisonous to ingest. Make cold compresses with witch hazel for painful hemorrhoids, varicose veins, or other skin inflammation and bruises. Take a witch hazel tincture, add fifteen drops to a small bowl of warm water, immerse a clean soft washcloth in the solution, and leave it soaking for five minutes. Wring out the washcloth and lay it on the affected area.

As an astringent, witch hazel works well for drying sores, diaper rash, and poison oak and ivy. Use witch hazel tincture (five drops to eight ounces water) if you want to avoid the isopropyl alcohol.

Apple Cider Skin Toner

This recipe utilizes apple cider vinegar, which should become one of your household mainstays. Many people assume—incorrectly—that vinegar will be irritating to skin, but it's actually quite the opposite as it neutralizes pH and softens skin. Apple cider vinegar will become one of your most-loved beauty fixes. To create a skin-soothing facial toner, just mix one-part water and one-part vinegar and apply to a cotton swab or soft clean cloth to wipe gently over a clean face.

Island Paradise Body Whip

Put one cup of coconut oil into a medium-sized bowl. Using a hand mixer and a whisk attachment, mix the oil until it reaches a soft, whipped-cream-like consistency. Add four drops of an essential oil with a scent you love into the mix and give it a last whip. Get in the bathtub naked and lather all over with the aromatic blend, then ease down into the water and just soak. Doesn't it feel luxurious?

Lavender Love Massage Bars

Massage bars should look, smell, and feel luxurious. Cocoa butter is beloved for its delicious chocolate scent.

I also recommend shea butter or mango butter as other options, for they are also sumptuous. You will need:

- ⫸ 3 ounces cocoa butter
- ⫸ 3 ounces beeswax
- ⫸ 3 ounces almond oil
- ⫸ 1 teaspoon of lavender essential oil
- ⫸ soap bar molds (available at all craft stores)

Slowly heat the beeswax, almond oil, and cocoa butter in a double boiler over low heat until just melted, then remove from heat. Add essential oil when mixture has cooled slightly and stir it in well. Pour into soap molds and cool until hardened, approximately two hours. Place in freezer for a few minutes before popping the bars out of the molds. To use, rub massage bar on the skin—the warmth of the skin immediately melts the bar. Package your handmade massage bar in a pretty lined basket and give it as a thoughtful gift.

Calming Balm: Bay Leaf

Any body oil or herbal oil can be turned into a salve with the addition of beeswax. The ratio for a salve is three ounces coconut oil to one ounce of beeswax. If you have a bay laurel tree nearby, pick some fresh leaves, or you can go to your spice rack and take three bay leaves from the jar. Grind the dried leaves in your mortar and pestle until broken up into fine little pieces. Set aside a fourth whole leaf. Use a double boiler to heat the oil and wax until completely melted. Test the viscosity of your salve by pouring a dab onto a cold plate. If you want the salve to have a denser texture, you will need to add more wax, and now is the time to do it. If satisfied with the consistency, pour off into jars to cool. Balms are simply salves with the addition of essential oils. Add two drops of eucalyptus essential oil and two drops of lemon oil while the mix is still warm. Sprinkle in the finely crushed bay laurel into the mix, stir well, and seal to preserve the aroma. Bay Leaf Balm will have a wonderfully calming effect anytime you use it and can be rubbed on your temples when you need to destress. I recommend Sunday night baths where you slather on the balm before stepping into a hot bath. Take a washcloth and massage your skin, then lie back and relax for twenty minutes. When you drain the tub, your stress will also empty out and you can start your week afresh, ready to handle anything that comes your way.

Rosemary Lavender Serenity Salve

- ❧ ½ cup rosemary essential oil
- ❧ ¼ cup lavender essential oil
- ❧ ¼ cup coconut oil
- ❧ 4 tablespoons beeswax

Combine the rosemary essential oils and the coconut oil. Heat the oil and wax together until the wax melts completely. Pour into a clean, dry jar. When the mixture has cooled a little but has not yet set, add the lavender essential oil, which is also an antiseptic, and stir gently.

Seal the jar and store in a cabinet to use anytime you scratch yourself working in the garden or want to renew and soften your hands and feet after a lot of house or yard work. Another note, use it on the outside of your skin and it will work wonders, but if a cut is deep, don't get it inside the wound. Let your physician handle that. Rosemary is a miracle plant for healing; in combination with the lavender, this power duo will restore your spirit along with your skin.

Tranquility Touch Massage Oil Blend

Sandalwood, lavender, and clary sage create a deeply soothing blend with a sensuous scent. Gather the following elements:

- ≫ ¼ cup of apricot or almond oil as a carrier oil
- ≫ 2 tablespoons jojoba oil
- ≫ 15 drops sandalwood essential oil
- ≫ 15 drops lavender essential oil
- ≫ 5 drops clary sage essential oil

Measure each oil into a dark-colored, sealable bottle. Carefully cap the bottle and gently shake until the oils are blended together. Shake well each time before using; store the bottle in a dark cupboard or shelf. Before using it on yourself or a loved one, you can warm it by putting the sealed bottle in a cup of warm water and letting it set there for five minutes. Many a masseuse pours the oil into her palms and lets it warm with her own body heat. Either way, warming your massage oil adds to the relaxation factor.

Light My Fire DIY Massage Candles

Making massage candles is very similar to making any other type of candle in a pot, tin, or can. I recommend using soy wax as it is soooo gentle on the skin. Soy is also nice and soft, so it melts easily and stays together in a puddle after melting and can be reused by us thrifty crafters. If you have an allergy to soy (and it won't irritate your skin unless you have a soy allergy), you can use beeswax instead, which is very widely used. (For example, it is in nearly every single Burt's Bees product.) It is the addition of the additional oils that prevents it from hardening again and enables your skin to absorb it. Essential oils or cosmetic-grade fragrance oils are also added to create a soothing atmosphere. All soap-making fragrances that are natural as well as soy candle safe are perfect choices for scenting your massage candles. Try the basic directions below to make your first candle. For every three ounces of wax, you'll add one ounce of liquid oil and one-quarter ounce of fragrance. I suggest making two candles in four-ounce metal tins as a step on the way to mastering this craft.

You will need these elements:

- 2 ounces sweet almond oil or vitamin E oil
- 6 ounces high quality soy wax

➽ Half an ounce essential oil

➽ 2 4-ounce metal tins

➽ 2 6-inch candle wicks

Directions

1. Melt the soy wax into the sweet almond oil or vitamin E oil in a double boiler over simmering water.

2. Add the essential oils and stir gently to avoid bubbling or spilling.

3. Once the wax has cooled somewhat but is still melted enough to pour, place the wicks in your containers and pour the wax.

4. Allow several hours for the candles to set and harden.

5. Trim the wicks to one-quarter of an inch above the top of each candle, and they're ready to use.

Sensual Scents for Massage Candles

Traditionally, these oils are considered to have aphrodisiac properties; besides that, they simply smell wonderful on your skin and in your home. Just burning the candles will be magical!

➽ Amber

➽ Cedarwood

➽ Clary sage

➽ Jasmine

➽ Neroli

➽ Patchouli

➽ Rose

➽ Sandalwood

➽ Vanilla

➽ Ylang-ylang

➽ Cinnamon

➽ Vetiver

Ageless Skin Spa Facial

You will notice that many an herbalist appears ageless. There is a good reason for this; we manifest a lot of joy in our lives, including creating potions to take excellent care of our skin for goddess-like youthfulness.

Combine these oils in a sealable dark blue bottle

- 2 ounces sweet almond as base oil
- 2 drops chamomile essential oil
- 2 drops rosemary essential oil
- 2 drops lavender essential oil

Shake very thoroughly and your potion is now ready to use.

Clean your skin with warm water, then gently daub your face with the mixture. You can also make a salve or balm using my recipe if you want to turn the clock backwards. Prepare to be asked for your beauty secrets a lot.

Herbal Enchantment

Here is a concise guide to the enchanted realm of herbs, essences, plants, and plant properties.

- **Benzoin** can be used for purification, prosperity, work success, mental acuity, and memory.
- **Camphor** can be used for healing, divining the future, curbing excess, especially romantic obsessions, and to cool a surfeit of sexuality.

➤ **Cinnamon** refreshes and directs spirituality. It is also a protection herb and handy for healing, money, love, lust, personal power, and success with work and creative projects.

➤ **Clove** is good for bringing money to you, for protection, for your love life, and for helping to evade and deter negative energies.

➤ **Copal** should be used for love, purification, and consecration.

➤ **Frankincense** is another spiritual essence that purifies, consecrates, and protects.

➤ **Lavender** is a plant for happiness, peace, true love, long life, and chastity, and it is an excellent purifier that aids with sleep.

➤ **Myrrh** has been considered since ancient times to be deeply sacred. It aids personal spirituality, heals and protects, and can help ward off negative spirits and energies.

➤ **Nutmeg** is a lucky herb that promotes good health and prosperity and encourages loyalty and fidelity in relationships.

➤ **Patchouli** stimulates and grounds while engendering both sensuality and fertility. It also supports personal wealth and security.

➤ **Peppermint** is an herb of purification, healing, and love. It supports relaxation, freedom from anxiety, and sleep as it helps to increase psychic powers.

➤ **Rosemary** is good for purification, protection, healing, relaxation, and intelligence. It attracts

love and sensuality, helps with memory, and can
keep you youthful.

⫸ **Sage** brings wisdom, purification, protection,
health, and a long life. It is very useful for
dispelling negative vibrations and cleansing, and
it can help make your wishes come true.

⫸ **Sandalwood** is a mystical, healing, protective
essence that helps attract the objects of your hopes
and desires as well as dispersing negative energies
and spirits.

⫸ **Star Anise** is a lucky herb that aids divination
and psychism.

⫸ **Tonka Bean** brings courage and draws love and
money to you.

⫸ **Vanilla** brings love and enriches your
mental capacity.

⫸ **Wood Aloe** is good for dressing or anointing
talismans and amulets you want to use
for protection.

Miracle Mint Foot Therapy

After a long day at the office, hiking, or
even dancing at your drum circle, our
feet get "dog tired." This pagan pick-me-
up will soon have you out and about,
feeling fresh and fabulous.

You need:

⫸   Mortar and pestle

➽ 3 tablespoons coconut oil, softened in a small bowl

➽ 1 teaspoon vinegar, either white or apple cider vinegar

➽ 3 drops mint essential oil

➽ Handful of fresh mint leaves, crushed

Place the coconut oil paste in the bowl and fold in the crushed mint leaves. Grind the mint leaves into the coconut thoroughly with your mortar and pestle. Add in the vinegar and the essential oil. Stir those in, then spoon the mixture into a small jar and place it in your freezer for five minutes. Sit in the side of the tub and gently massage the mint mix into your feet, giving every toe and heel lots of loving attention. Take your time, as your feet do so much work all day, every day. When you are satisfied, rinse your feet clean in the shower, carefully making sure not to slip on the coconut oil. Now, you deserve to put your feet up and just enjoy life.

Rosemary and Thyme: A Rejuvenation Retreat

All of us get worn down due to the sheer busyness of life. Oftentimes when we feel depleted, we get a little sad, too. To rid yourself of negative emotions, try this purification bath. Draw a warm bath at noon when the sun is at its healing peak, then add the following essential oils into the water as it flows from the faucet.

➽ Two drops rosemary for calm

➽ Two drops peppermint for stimulation

❧   Three drops lavender for energetic cleansing

❧   Three drops thyme to relieve mental exhaustion

As you soak and steam, repeat this prayer four times:

> *Sadness, I release you—goodbye.*
> *Fatigue, I release you—goodbye.*
> *I greet this day anew. My life is now renewed.*
> *Blessed be me, so mote it be.*

Spa Feng Shui: Sauna Serenity

The Scandinavians make sure their saunas have bunches of wonderfully fragrant silver birch branches hanging nearby that they can use to gently brush their skin to stimulate circulation. This sauna practice is deeply relaxing and can be a marvelous communal experience. No wonder Denmark is the happiest place on earth!

You can emulate this by hanging herbs from your shower rod or above your bathtub. This infuses the aromatic oils into the air as soon as the steam hits the herbs. We recommend bunches of lavender for tranquility and eucalyptus to aid with colds and congestion. A muslin bag filled with dried orange rind and dressed with orange essential oil will lift depression. Rosemary can help you process sadness and grief and activates your memory. A big bag of mint leaves is a major mood booster and sends concentration levels soaring. After a few uses, these herbs can be dried by laying them on a baking sheet and setting them aside in a cool dry place for two weeks. Once dry, tie into a bundle with twine and add it to a bonfire for the high holidays. Enjoy the holy and sweet-smelling smoke as it ascends into the heavens!

CHAPTER FIVE

Teas, Tinctures, Oxymels, and *More!*

. . . .

All herbalists have one thing in common with the British—they believe a good pot of tea can fix 'most anything. And it is true—heartache, headaches, and all manner of ills seem to evaporate in the steam that rises from the spout of the kettle. With a handful of herbs and a cauldron-full of witchy wisdom, big healing can result from a small cup of tea. Once you have the knack of that, you can also brew up simples, digestives, tisanes, tonics, tinctures, and many other concoctions that can be created right at home. This is one of the most delightful DIY aspects of herbal healing, the fact that these recipes are usually easy enough as long as you have the proper ingredients. They can be enjoyed alone and make all the difference after a long day at the office, and they can also be shared to great effect. Bottled and hand labeled, these potions also make significant gifts that will be long remembered for their thoughtfulness as well as for the delight and comfort received. Prepare to brew up much joy.

Simples

Teas brewed from a single herb are commonly called simples, a lovely phrase from olden times. Experience has taught me that simples often have the most potency; the purity of that single plant essence can come through undiluted. This book contains a plentitude of helpful, healing, and tasty simples you can brew, but yarrow is one you should brew regularly. Boil one pint of spring water. Combine with a half-ounce of dried yarrow in your favorite crockery pot. Steep for ten minutes and strain with a nonmetallic implement, such as an inexpensive bamboo strainer or cheesecloth. Sweeten with honey; clover honey intensifies the positivity of this potion and makes it a supremely lucky drink. Yarrow brings courage and nourishes a strong heart as it is a major medicinal; it is also useful for fever. All these aspects make yarrow one of the most strengthening of all simples.

Two Simples Every Woman Should Know

Red raspberry leaf and chasteberry are each simples that are invaluable for women's health and healing. Raspberry leaf taken as an infusion can *prevent* menstrual cramps for most women. Take a teaspoon to a small handful (depending on severity of cramps experienced) and steep covered in freshly boiled water for ten minutes. Head those cramps off at the pass by drinking one cup per day for a week before you expect your cycle to begin. (For *severe* cramps, take this herb every day of the month!) This herb actually has a pleasant flavor and can be used to make caffeine-free ice tea or sweet tea (but if you are having cramps on the day you plan to drink it, its healing effect will work better if you drink it warm). Raspberry leaf combines well both in taste and effect with many other common simples, such as chamomile or mint, so you can experiment with flavor combinations...or even invent your own custom moon time tea!

Why does raspberry leaf have this wonderful effect? An aromatherapist of my acquaintance tells me that in pharmacological research, this plant has been shown to improve the tone and condition of the uterus! Which is why it is *also* the number one simple an expectant mother ought to include in her regimen. At least one strong cup daily is recommended to support your body in the process of creation during every month of pregnancy.

Chasteberry (also known as "Vitex" from its scientific name, *Vitex agnus castus*), is the number one simple for the power surges known as hot flashes frequently experienced by ladies in their middle years. The part used is the berries; simmer a couple of teaspoons low in a cup or two of water after bringing the water to a boil, making sure to cover the pot so as not to lose the medicinal volatile essence. This herb tastes medicinal but not terrible and can be combined with any mild herbal tea for flavor. If you prefer convenience, either chasteberry or raspberry leaf can be purchased in capsules, though it is a bit more costly to take them that way.

Always choose organic medicinal herbs when you can find (and afford) them, not only to be kind to Mother Earth but because their healing effects are stronger.

Black and Green Tea

Use black tea for an upset tummy and diarrhea. Green tea strengthens the immune system, and you can reuse lightly moistened tea bags to stanch minor cuts or calm insect bites.

White Tea

White tea, green tea, and black tea are all made from the leaves of *Camellia sinensis*. White tea is made from the youngest leaves of the plant; it is a naturally sweet brew and has less caffeine than green or black tea. It is also rich in antioxidants and is recommended for reducing "bad" cholesterol and improving artery health. White tea is a little costly but a good choice for health and flavor.

Jasmine Tea Will Bring You Joy

Jasmine tea is a delightful concoction and can create an aura of bliss and conviviality. It is available at any grocer or purveyor of organic goods, but homegrown is even better. Brew a cup of jasmine tea and let it cool. Add two parts lemonade and drink the mixture with a good friend. Jasmine is a vine and represents the intertwining of people. You will be more bonded to anyone with whom you share this sweet ritual. This is also a tonic in which you can indulge alone. I recommend brewing up a batch every Monday, or "Moon Day," to ensure that each week is filled with joyfulness.

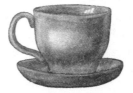

Tea-lepathy

The humble dandelion, abhorred by lawn keepers everywhere, hides its might very well. Dandelion root tea can call upon the spirit of anyone whose advice you might need. Simply place a freshly brewed simple using this herbal root on your bedroom altar or nightstand. Before you sleep, say the name of your spirit helper aloud seven times. In a dream or vision, the spirit will visit you and answer all your questions. During medieval times, this spell was used to find hidden treasure. Chaucer, who was well-versed in astrology and other metaphysics, advised this tried-and-true tea.

Steeped in Wisdom

Different kinds of tea can combine to make a powerful concoction. A pot of your favorite grocer's black tea can become a magical potion with the addition of a thin slice of ginger root, a pinch of dried chamomile, and the same amount of peppermint tea. This ambrosial brew can calm any storm at home or at work.

Herbal tea nourishes the soul, heals the body, and calms the mind. Try these:

- **Blackberry** leaf tea reduces mood swings, and it evens glucose levels, aiding in weight management. This miraculous herbal even helps circulation and such issues as inflammation and varicose veins. It is helpful to cancer patients and is believed to be a preventative.

- **Cardamom** is a favorite of expectant mothers everywhere as it calms nausea and morning sickness; this fragrant East Indian spice is excellent for digestion and clears and cleans your mouth and throat. Anyone who likes cinnamon will love cardamom.

- **Nettle** raises your energy level, boosts the immune system, and is packed with iron and vitamins.

- **Fennel** is awakening and uplifting and is excellent for digestion and cleansing. Fennel is also is a natural breath freshener.

- **Catnip** is one of the witchiest of teas; it is not only grown as fun for your feline familiar. Catnip is a gentle but potent sleep-inducer. At the first inkling of a sore throat or impending cold, drink a warm cup of catnip tea and head off to bed and you will awaken feeling much better. Catnip soothes the nervous system and can safely help get a restless child off to sleep.

- **Echinacea** lends an increased and consistent sense of well-being and prevents colds and flu.

It is a very powerful immune booster. Take a simmered low echinacea root tea for up to two weeks at a time to jumpstart your immune system; an ounce a week of echinacea tincture will also serve if convenience is needed. (The tincture is rather medicinal tasting, so best dilute it in a cup of juice or your favorite plant-based beverage.)

⫸ **Ginger Root** calms and cheers while aiding digestion, fighting nausea, and helping fend off coughs and sore throats.

⫸ **Dandelion Root** grounds and centers as it provides many minerals and nutrients. This wonderful weed is also a cleanser and a wholly natural detoxifier and liver tonic.

A Soothing Sip

Here is a soothing sip that can uplift your spirits anytime and serves to ward off chills. This combination of herbs helps to bring about letting go of sorrows, worries, and doubts and reignites feelings of self-love.

Stir the following together in a clean cauldron:

⫸ One ounce dried rosehips

⫸ One ounce dried hibiscus flowers

⫸ Two ounces dried mint

⫸ One tablespoon dried ginger root, coarsely chopped or ground

Combine the herbs, pour into a colored jar, and seal the lid tightly. When you are ready to brew a soothing tea, pour hot water over the herbs: one cup of hot water to each two teaspoons of tea. While this steeps for five minutes, write down any thoughts or fears from which you need to release yourself on a small piece of paper. Now say each one aloud, then chant, "Begone!" following each. After this letting-go ritual, burn the paper with sage in a small cauldron on your altar. As you sip the tea, enjoy your renewed sense of self and peace of mind.

Gardener's Tea

As you now know, tilling the back forty, weeding, and harvesting your herbs and veggies is a huge amount of work. It is one of life's greatest joys, without doubt, but nevertheless, many a sore back or aching knees have come to pass as result of a thriving garden. All the more reason for tea that revives, refreshes, and offers relief to aching joints. From your store of dried herbs, gather these:

- ❧ 2 parts echinacea root
- ❧ 2 parts chamomile flowers
- ❧ 1 part mint
- ❧ 1 part anise seed
- ❧ 1 part thyme

A nice hot cup of this remedy will have you jumping back into the garden to plant more of all the herbs that comprise this delightful tea. Ahhhh, sit back and enjoy. You deserve it!

Peachy Keen Cooler

Not every herbal tea works well over ice, but this one will have your family and friends clamoring for more. Gather a palmful of each of these dried herbs:

- ➤ 1 part each of lemon verbena and lemon balm
- ➤ 1 part each of mint leaves, chamomile flowers, and hibiscus flowers
- ➤ 2 cups peach juice
- ➤ 1 lemon

Brew the herbs to yield six cups and let cool to room temperature. Pour into a large pitcher and add the peach juice until the pitcher is two-thirds full. Give it a good stir, then add in enough ice cubes to fill the vessel. Slice the lemon and lay on top. Serve, sit back, and let the compliments begin. This convivial concoction is ideal for special summer occasions such as the midsummer celebration of the solstice or longest day of the year.

A Tincture in Time Saves Nine

Herbal tinctures, which are concentrated extracts of the herbs, are more expensive but last longer and provide a higher dose of the herb. We keep a tincture of echinacea and goldenseal in the house year-round. At the first sign of a cold or cough, a few drops go into herbal teas and hot lemon and honey toddies. A hot toddy is traditionally made with hot water, lemon, sugar or honey, and liquor such as brandy, but it doesn't have to be alcoholic to be medicinal. Fresh ginger and garlic are great for adding to home remedies, particularly for colds; just chop finely or grate and add to teas and toddies.

Ginger Is Your Go-To for Getting Better Quickly

Ginger is indicated for a sore throat and is a good addition to a hot toddy for cold symptoms. Ginger is known to alleviate indigestion, general nausea, upset tummy, morning sickness, and stomach flu. Ginger tea has a very pleasant taste, and you can either buy it in tea bags or gently simmer slices of fresh ginger root on a low burner to make the tea yourself; I recommend using the fresh ginger root for maximum taste and potency. Arthritic pain can be treated with ginger, too; three to four grams (about a tenth of an ounce) daily is recommended, and ginger can also be taken either in capsules or as tinctures.

First Aid Tip

When you are getting over an illness, eat light broths, either vegetable or chicken. Broths are easy to digest, saving your body's energy for recovery.

Garlic Is Good for Everything

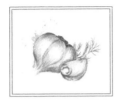

Garlic is well-known for its ability to protect against infection and should be used regularly (to taste!) in your cooking. It is also known to reduce cholesterol levels and can be helpful in lowering blood pressure. Rich in vitamins A, B, and C, garlic is an excellent source of minerals: selenium, iodine, potassium, iron, calcium, zinc, and magnesium. The active component in garlic is allicin, a sulfur compound produced when garlic is chopped, chewed, or bruised. It is powerful as an antibiotic and helps the body inhibit the ability of germs to grow and reproduce. When preparing garlic, cut or crush the cloves, then let the garlic rest for ten minutes before cooking or eating to allow the allicin to develop. Garlic is cited as therapeutic for the treatment of many health conditions, such as both high *and* low blood pressure, heart problems, and asthma, as well as being acknowledged as an anti-cancer agent and a preventative for colds and other infections.

Although garlic pills are available, raw garlic is just as effective and considerably cheaper. For a simple garlic tonic to guard against colds or just to boost your general health, crush a couple of cloves and add a tablespoon of olive oil. Taking a spoonful of garlic in olive oil works well if you don't like the taste or are fearful of unappealingly garlicky breath.

At the onset of an earache, take a peeled clove, wrap it in a little fabric such as cheesecloth, and stick it in your sore ear, taking care not to insert it too deeply.

Leave it there overnight, and you will feel some relief by the morning.

Grapefruit Seed Extract

Grapefruit seed extract is a powerful substance. It is a powerful general immune tonic that can help a wide spectrum of conditions ranging from healing cuts to respiratory viral illnesses. It is very strong and should never be taken undiluted nor used neat in a topical application. I use it when afflicted with a stomach bug with symptoms of vomiting and diarrhea. Take five to ten drops in eight ounces of juice or tea, which will help disguise its strong bitter taste; grapefruit or other citrus juices disguise its bitterness particularly effectively. For a child, give three to five drops in five ounces of juice or tea. These doses should be taken morning and evening and will clear up a stomach bug pretty quickly. After taking grapefruit seed extract, also take some acidophilus, either in natural yogurt or in the form of a tablet. This will restore your "friendly" intestinal flora to a healthy, balanced state. Grapefruit seed extract is also recommended as a gingivitis treatment: add three drops to five ounces of water and use as a mouthwash—rinse and spit, but try not to swallow!

For an effective dandruff cure, add five drops of grapefruit seed extract to your usual dollop of hair shampoo and massage it into the scalp.

For a wart or cyst, apply a drop of grapefruit seed extract daily directly to the affected spot and cover with a bandage.

Aloe Vera Juice and Gel

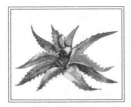

As a topical application, aloe vera gel is great for all kinds of burns, including sunburn. It has been shown to have therapeutic value in the healing of skin lesions caused by psoriasis. The juice is a great general tonic as it is recommended as an aid to digestion, a stimulus for intestinal health, and a gentle colon cleanse. Aloe vera is one of the few vegetarian sources of vitamin B12 and contains nineteen amino acids, twenty minerals, and twelve vitamins, all of which have a beneficial effect on general health. Drinking four to eight ounces daily diluted in juice or taken neat is recommended, but even just a couple of times a week will be beneficial.

Baking Soda Basics

Baking soda is great in a bath if your skin is irritated, especially if the cause is poison oak or ivy, as the soda will help dry up wet blisters as well as greatly reducing the itch. Applying a baking soda and water paste to the site of a bee sting or other insect bite will neutralize the pain and itch. Just remove the actual stinger first, and then smooth on the baking soda paste for instant relief.

A headache can be treated with a teaspoon of baking soda dissolved in a cup of warm water with ¼ cup of freshly squeezed lemon juice.

Last but not least, whiten your teeth and freshen your breath by brushing with baking soda and water.

Your Apple a Day: Simple Apple Cider Vinegar

This easy-peasy recipe will result in one of the most useful items in your pantry, one which can be used not only in your cookery and as a daily health drink, but as a household cleanser, skin and facial toner, hair rinse, and dozens of other excellent uses. Hippocrates, the founding father of medicine in ancient Greece, taught that he depended on two medicinal tonics, honey and vinegar. Apple cider vinegar lowers cholesterol and blood pressure and helps strengthen bones. Best of all, this preparation costs mere pennies to make as you are using only the cores and peels from the apples. Bake a couple of pies while you brew up a tonic to boost health. When you add herbs to vinegar, you are enhancing their healing power synergistically for the best of both worlds. All you need is:

- ❯ cores and peels of 8 organic apples
- ❯ 2 tablespoons of honey
- ❯ 1 quart of water

Cut up the apple cores and peels into smaller pieces and spoon them into a wide-mouthed canning jar. Pour in enough water to cover the fruit, then spoon in the honey and stir well. Cover the jar with either a clean paper towel or waxed paper and place a rubber band tightly around the neck of the jar. Place on a dark shelf in your cupboard or work area and leave it for two weeks. After a fortnight, strain the liquid and remove and discard the compostable solids that remain. then return the liquid to the jar and secure the cover with the rubber band again. Put it back on the shelf. making sure to stir it daily. After one month, taste a spoonful; if the acidity and flavor is to your taste, transfer it to a dark bottle with a sealable top. Vinegar from the fermented apples will corrode metal lids, so a pretty bottle with a cork is the best option.

Make Your Own Herbal Vinegar

If you love everything about lavender, you may well want to create your own lavender vinegar. Many herbs make excellent vinegars, so pay attention to which ones especially appeal to you as you go about your gardening. The more herbs you pack into the jar, the higher the mineral content in your vinegar, which makes it more flavorful and healthful. Once you have your own apple cider vinegar or a premade organic variety you and your family love, pick an herb you know works for you and pack a quart canning jar as full of that herb as you can. Pour room temperature apple cider vinegar to cover, then cover it with paper and rubber bands and pop on a dark corner shelf for six weeks, giving the jar a shake once a week. At the end of the infusion period, strain out any remaining compostable twigs or stems. Store your herb vinegar in a colored bottle and add a pretty label. These make wonderful gifts, so I recommend you either create or acquire a set of labels for all your herbal brews.

Blessings on a Budget

Instead of composting all the herbs, twigs, and stems from your brews, you can store them in a burlap or muslin sack and allow them to dry. Keep stuffing in twigs of lavender, rosemary, mint, and all the leftover aromatic plant material until you have a big bag. On some special evening, burn it in your fireplace or an outdoor bonfire, and it will be like a gigantic incense burner with the lovely scents wafting from the flames. And the best part? It's 100 percent free!

Garden Alchemy: Perfect Plants for DIY Vinegars

The leaves and stalks of the following plants are very good for making herbal vinegars: apple mint, basil, catnip, garlic, mustard, orange mint, peppermint, rosemary, spearmint, thyme, and yarrow.

Dill and fennel seeds work very well, as do lemon and orange peels.

The flowers of bee balm, chives, goldenrod, lavender, and yarrow make for delicate herbed vinegars.

Roots also infuse nicely into herbal vinegars—the best are dandelion, chicory, ginger, garlic, mugwort, and burdock.

Old Thyme Tincture: Medicinal Herbal Vinegar

Every kitchen garden should be strewn with thyme plantings, fragrantly growing amongst the flagstones in the path as well as in the rows of herbs, filling the air with their magnificent scent and elegant beauty. You will need to keep a plentitude growing and several bunches drying in a dark corner of your panty at all times, as this plant makes a mighty fine tincture with many medicinal uses. I also suggest you start gathering together some supplies: clean muslin or cheesecloth, several colored glass bottles, and an assortment of canning jars with lids for storing your handiwork. For this tincture, take one of the larger jars and the following ingredients:

- ⁂ 1¼ cup dried thyme leaves
- ⁂ 2 cups apple cider vinegar

Put the dried thyme in the jar and carefully pour the vinegar inside. Stir well and seal. Place on a dark shelf and make sure to shake it every day. At the end of the one month, strain through muslin. Compost the thyme residue in your garden and store the tincture in a pretty glass jar.

Having this herbal helper around will come in handy for mouthwashes, hair rinses, and ritual baths, and you can even rub it on achy joints and sore muscles. For a cup of thyme tea, add one teaspoon of the tincture to a cup of hot water, then add a teaspoon of honey, stir, and enjoy.

Bee Healthy with Miracle Salve

Thyme in the garden attracts bees, and honey made by these "thymely bees" is highly sought after. If you can come by this rarity, get as much as you can as it is redolent with Mother Nature's love and enchantment. The ancient Greeks prized thyme honey very highly not only as a delicacy at the table but as a miracle salve to heal everything: the stomach, aches and pains, and even wounds. Hippocrates swore by it!

Luxuriating in Lavender

Lavender is hard *not* to grow; once your seedlings and young plants have been established, they will bush out and produce loads of scented stalks, flowers, and seeds. This bounty will become your source for teas, tinctures, bath salts, and infusions. For tea, the rule of thumb is one teaspoon dried lavender flowers to one cup boiling water to aid tummy trouble, headache, aches, and insomnia and even help calm the mind. You can easily amp up the therapeutic power of your brew by adding any of these excellent herbs: dried yarrow, St. John's Wort, or chamomile.

Here is a simple and streamlined way to infuse lavender:

Pour a heaping tablespoon of lavender blossoms into a bowl of hot water, then drape a towel over your head and breathe in the aromatic fumes to deal with respiratory issues, coughs, colds, headaches, stuffy sinuses, and nervous tension. You will come away feeling renewed, and your kitchen will smell like the heavens above. Afterwards, you can use the water in your morning bath, to wash your face or hands, or to freshen your sink garbage disposal; grinding up the flowers refreshes that hardworking kitchen appliance.

Lavandula Tranquility Tincture

This cure-all should be kept on hand at all times for soothing the skin, the stomach, and anything in need of comfort. I have even seen it used to stanch bleeding in small cuts. You need:

- ⇛ dried lavender
- ⇛ dried calendula
- ⇛ clear quart jar with lid
- ⇛ cheesecloth
- ⇛ dark glass jar for storage
- ⇛ 2 cups distilled water
- ⇛ 1 cup clear alcohol such as vodka or Everclear

Fill your clear quart jar to the halfway point with the dried lavender and calendula. Pour in the alcohol, also to the halfway point. Add in the two cups of water, seal the lid securely, and shake for a few minutes until it seems well mixed. Store in a dark cupboard for one month, shaking once a day. After thirty days, strain through cheesecloth into the dark glass storage jar and screw the lid on tightly. The lavender leavings will make lovely compost, and the liquid tincture will soon prove itself indispensable in your household.

Pantry Power—Plant Infusions That Heal and Help

Many enthusiasts enjoy several cups a day of their favorite herbal infusion, which is a large portion of herb brewed for at least four hours and perhaps as long as ten. I recommend placing one cup of the dried herb into a quart canning jar and filling it with freshly boiled water. After the steeping, strain with a nonmetallic type of strainer such as cheesecloth or bamboo. Herbal infusions can be made with the leaves and fruits, which provide the healing aspects of this type of comforting brew. Many favorite herbs from your kitchen garden contain minerals, antioxidants, and phytochemicals, including the list herein.

What do you need to attend in your life now? This list of herbs and associations can be your guide; one of the smartest ways to approach this methodology is to brew right before bedtime so you will awaken to a freshly infused herb. Some of the most popular herbs and fruits used to create infusions are as follows:

- 🌿 Anise Seeds & Leaves: soothe cramps and aches

- 🌿 Caraway Seeds: aid in romantic issues, help with colic

- 🌿 Catnip Leaves: make women even more attractive

- Chamomile Flowers: help with sleep, good for abundance

- Dandelion Leaves: make wishes come true

- Echinacea: makes the body strong

- Ginseng Root: increases men's vigor

- Nettle Leaves: lung function, hex breaking

- Peppermint Leaves: clearing tummy discomfort, cleansing

- Pine Needles: increase skin health as well as financial health

- Rose Hip Fruit: packed with vitamin C and can halt colds and flu

- Sage Leaves: purify energy, antibiotic

- Skullcap Leaves: prevent insomnia and soothe nerves

- St. John's Wort Flowers: antidepressant

- Thyme Leaves: antiseptic, protectant

- Yarrow Flowers: reduce fever, bring courage and good luck

Liquid Love: Spicy Cinnamon Liqueur

This popular beverage gives peppy energy and can also be a love potion. These few ingredients can lead to a lifetime of love and devotion:

- ⤜ 1 cup vodka

- ⤜ 2 whole cloves

- ⤜ 1 teaspoon ground coriander seed

- ⤜ 1 cinnamon stick

- ⤜ 1 cup simple sugar syrup

Pour the vodka into a bowl and add in the herbs; cover and place in a cupboard for two weeks. Strain and filter until the result is clear liquid. Clean the canning jar and dry it thoroughly, then put the clear liquid back in. Add the simple syrup and place back on the shelf for a week. Store this in a dark-colored bottle that seals; you now have liquid love! You can drink it "neat" on its own or add this to hot chocolate, water, tea, or milk for a delightful drink to share with your loved one.

DIY Digestive Elixir

You can make simple syrup, a base for any liqueur, in five short minutes by boiling a cup of sugar in a half cup of water. The method above can be used to create distinctive after-dinner drinks and digestives with angelica, anise, bergamot, hyssop, all mints, fennel, and perhaps the most special of all, violets. To your health!

Mulled Medieval Merriment for Holidays & More

Start this special mixture brewing by pouring a cup of unfiltered sweet apple cider into a big pot. Go for organic fruit at the farmer's market, but it is even better if you can make it yourself from apples you have gathered or harvested. Take a bottle of your favorite low-cost red wine and gently heat with the cider in a medium saucepan on a low flame. Add sugar, cinnamon, and cloves to your taste, but at least a tablespoon of each, and stir every six minutes. Notice how your entire home fills with the spicy sweetness of merriment. After thirty minutes, your brew should be ready to serve.

CHAPTER SIX

Your Healing Pantry—DIY Pickles, Jams, Canned Preserves, and Liqueurs to Enjoy All Year 'Round

. . . .

We are experiencing a witchy renaissance here in the early years of the twenty-first century. So many of us, myself included, can get whelmed just thinking about how to handle the stress, strain, and over busyness of modern life. My one surefire approach to managing worry and a wildly racing monkey mind is to head to the kitchen. Brewing up a pot of herbal tea, a healing herbal brew, a spice-filled liqueur, or a floral tincture immediately relaxes me. Cooking up a healthy meal or putting up a batch of pickles or preserves, as my mom and aunties say, is enormously rewarding and will not only have you feeling better about yourself and the world, but also will also end up creating something delicious you can share. These homely magical arts are also a kind of witchcraft with a very important ingredient: love!

Cures from Your Kitchen

Many remedies can be made from what you have in the kitchen, from spices as well as other plants. Here are a few simple tried and tested recipes:

Nutmeg Milk

Grated nutmeg soothes diarrhea and upset tummies. Use a nutmeg grater to grate a small amount (about ⅛ teaspoon) into warmed milk (cow, soy, rice, or oat milk).

Cayenne Infusion

Use this pepper as a remedy for colds, coughs, sore throats, heartburn, hemorrhoids, and varicose veins, or as a digestive stimulant and to improve circulation. Make an infusion by adding ½ teaspoon cayenne powder to one cup boiled water. Dilute with two cups of hot water to make a more pleasant and palatable infusion. Add lemon and honey to taste. (Be careful; it will be spicy! If you don't enjoy hot spicy flavors, consider supplementing powdered cayenne in capsules.)

Easy Turmeric Detox

This spice is a natural antioxidant, antiseptic, and antibacterial. Turmeric is also detoxifying for the liver and curative for acne and common colds. It is a popular herb for decreasing inflammation at a system level in your body; this can soothe soreness in joints in a way that is deeper than mere symptomatic relief. Make a turmeric tea by adding a teaspoon of the powder to four cups of boiling water. Simmer over low heat until it dissolves, then add milk and honey to taste.

Cabbage Juice Curative

This commonplace vegetable is a fantastic antibacterial and anti-inflammatory. Cabbage can be used for stomach ulcers, arthritis, and swollen joints, or as a liver tonic. To create a cabbage tonic, dilute one part cabbage juice with two parts water. For swollen joints and arthritic pain, lightly crush a few green outer cabbage leaves with a rolling pin, then lay them over the afflicted area with the inner side of the leaf on your skin, secured with a bandage. Some prefer to boil the leaves, let them cool, and then apply. Going to bed with a cabbage bandage on is also good, giving the leaf time to work its magic.

Lemon Water

Use this citrus fruit for colds and infections. Add the fresh-squeezed juice to hot water with honey to taste. For a fast sore-throat curative, use unsweetened lemon juice with warm water as an antiseptic gargle.

Sun-Infused Flower Essences

For centuries, flower essences have been used to heal many infirmities (see list below). While the health food shop versions are handy, they are also very spendy. You can make your own flower essences at home. Start by making a mother essence—the most concentrated form of the essence—which can then be used to make stock bottles. The stock bottles are used to make dosing bottles for the most diluted form of the essence, which is what you actually take.

What you will need to make a sun-infused mother essence:

- ⇛ 3 quarts of fresh pure spring water or distilled water, 3 quarts

- ⇛ Clear glass 2½-quart mixing bowl

- ⇛ An 8-ounce sealable bottle made of dark green, blue, or green glass

- ⇛ Organic brandy or vodka

- ⇛ Freshly picked flowers specific to the malady being treated

- ⇛ Clean, dry cheesecloth for straining.

Ideally, you begin early in the morning and pick your chosen flowers by nine o'clock at the latest. This all ensures three hours of sunlight before the noon hour, after which the sunlight is less effective, or even draining.

Fill the bowl with the fresh water; to avoid touching them, place the flowers very carefully on the surface of the water using tweezers or chopsticks to gently add blooms until the water's surface is covered. Let the bowl sit in the sun for three to four hours or until the flowers begin to fade.

Now, delicately remove the flowers, being careful not to touch the water with your fingers. Fill your colored glass bottle with the strained flower essence water and top the other half off with the organic brandy or vodka (40 percent proof is advised to prolong the shelf life to three months if stored in a cool, dark cupboard). This is your mother tincture; label it with the date and the name of the flower, such as, "Rose Water, July 14, 2021." Use any remaining essence water to water the flowers you've been working with and murmur a prayer of gratitude for their beauty and healing power.

To make a stock bottle from your mother tincture, fill a one ounce (thirty ml) dropper bottle ¾ full of brandy, top it up with ¼ spring water, then add three drops of the mother tincture. This will last at least three months, enabling you to make lots of dosing bottles, which are the ones from which you actually take the flower essence.

To make the dosage bottle for any flower essence just add two or three drops of the stock bottle to another thirty ml dropper bottle of ¼ brandy and ¾ distilled water. Anytime, you need some of this gentle medicine, place four drops of this under your tongue or sip in a glass of water four times a day or as often as you feel the need. You can't overdose on flower remedies, though more frequent, rather than larger, doses are much more effective.

Flower essences mixed with one ounce (thirty ml) of pure spring water or distilled water can also be used to help the following conditions:

- ⋙ Addiction: *skullcap, agrimony*
- ⋙ Anger: *nettle, blue flag, chamomile*
- ⋙ Anxiety: *garlic, rosemary, aspen, periwinkle, lemon balm, white chestnut, gentian*
- ⋙ Bereavement: *honeysuckle*
- ⋙ Depression: *borage, sunflower, larch, chamomile, geranium, yerba santa, black cohosh, lavender, mustard*
- ⋙ Exhaustion: *aloe, yarrow, olive, sweet chestnut*
- ⋙ Fear: *poppy, mallow, ginger, peony, water lily, basil, datura*
- ⋙ Heartbreak: *heartsease, hawthorn, borage*
- ⋙ Lethargy: *aloe, thyme, peppermint*
- ⋙ Stress: *dill, echinacea, thyme, mistletoe, lemon balm*
- ⋙ Spiritual blocks: *oak, ginseng, lady's slipper*

Rose Hips: Mother Nature's Vitamins Growing from Flowers

Once a rose has bloomed and all petals have fallen away, the hip is ready to be picked. Ground rose hips are the best source of immune-boosting vitamin C; they contain 50 percent more vitamin C than oranges. One tablespoon provides more than the recommended daily adult allowance of sixty mg. The pulp from rose hips may be used in sauces or made into jelly. What a delicious way to ward off colds and ailments!

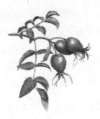

Rose hip

Blessed Batch of Pickles: A Garden in a Jar

This is a recipe handed down from generation to generation in my family. My mother was very proud of and famous for her pickles. This same cucumber recipe can be used to pickle almost any vegetable, including onions, peppers, squash, baby corn, green tomatoes, cauliflower, and anything else you might fancy. Growing your own dill will be a wonderful finishing touch. Gather:

- ❧ 3 dozen baby cucumbers (three to four inches long)

- ❧ 3 cups water

- ❧ 3 cups vinegar

- ❧ 6 tablespoons kosher salt

- ❧ 1 bunch fresh dill or ½ teaspoon dried dill per jar (you can use seed heads, leaves, and stems, too)

- ❧ ½ to 1 clove garlic per jar, blanched and sliced

- ❧ ½ tablespoon mustard seed per jar

≫ 2-quart Mason canning jars (or 6 one-pint jars), sterilized

Wash all the cucumbers using cool water. In a big stockpot, pour in the vinegar, three cups of water, and the kosher salt and bring to a boil. This is the brining liquid. In the bottom of a sterilized quart jar, place a generous layer of dill, a clove of garlic, and ½ tablespoon mustard seed. Pack the cucumbers vertically into the jar until half full, then add another layer of dill and fill the remainder of the jar with cucumbers. Fill all the jars in the exact same way, leaving a half-inch at the top for brine. After you have poured in the brining liquid, go ahead and seal the Mason jars. Place the jars in a boiling-water bath for fifteen minutes. Label once your pickle jars have cooled and store on a cool, dark shelf for two weeks to allow the flavor to develop.

Magical correspondences to draw from in labeling your fresh batch of pickles:

≫ Cucumber: healing, peace

≫ Vinegar: security, cleansing

≫ Dill: prosperity, safety, luck

≫ Garlic: protection, healing

≫ Salt: purification

Strawberry Fields Jam

July is one of the sweetest times to enjoy your garden, and strawberries are a harbinger of the good summertimes ahead. To make this lucky jam, you will need the following ingredients:

- 🐾 5 cups of strawberries
- 🐾 1 teaspoon unsalted butter
- 🐾 1¾ ounces powdered fruit pectin
- 🐾 7 cups granulated sugar
- 🐾 ½ cup fresh basil, chopped
- 🐾 9 clean and sterilized 1-pint canning jars

Macerate the strawberries in a big bowl. In a large pot, melt the butter, then pour in the crushed strawberries. Fold in the powdered pectin. Heat the mixture to a full boil over high heat, stirring constantly. Add in the sugar and bring to a full rolling boil again. Boil and stir for one more minute. Now, add in the chopped basil.

Remove the pot from heat and skim off any foam. Ladle the hot mixture into nine half-pint jars, leaving ¼-inch at the top. Look for and remove any air bubbles. If you need to fill in the jars, add in more hot jam mixture. Carefully wipe the jar rims, then seal the lids on the jars. Place jars into canner with simmering water, ensuring that they are completely covered with water. Bring to a boil; process for ten minutes. Remove jars and cool. Strawberries are widely regarded as an aphrodisiac, and basil brings money to your house. Making this "Love and Money Jam" will be a great gift to everyone in your household and anyone who is served this jolliest of jams.

Summer Sweet Blackberry Jam

Below is a tried-and-true recipe for a simple berry jam. Our family favorite is blackberries as the color of the jam is nearly as delicious as its taste when spread on warm toast. You'll need the following:

- ⫸ 2 cups blackberries (or try raspberries or strawberries)
- ⫸ 2 cups sugar
- ⫸ 2 teaspoons lemon juice
- ⫸ 1 slice of lemon rind
- ⫸ Apple slice
- ⫸ Canning jars and tongs

Crush the berries with a potato masher, softly, not too hard. Place all the ingredients in a stockpot and boil over high heat for five minutes, stirring the mixture to prevent it from sticking or burning. Reduce the heat to medium-high and continue to boil and stir. Remove any foam with a large spoon. After a half hour, the jam will begin to thicken up. If your jam is setting slowly, you can add more lemon juice or a slice of apple. Pectin, which is regularly used thicken jams and jellies, is made from apples. Thus, a slice of apple will serve the same purpose.

When the jam is ready, pour it into sterilized jars. The jars should be warm when the jam is added, so keep the sterilized articles in the oven, dishwasher, or canning water bath until you need them; ditto the lids and rings.

Make sure to leave a generous half-inch gap between the jam and the top of the jar—this is known as headspace in the world of jam. Place the lids on the jars and screw them on firmly.

Place the sealed jars into the water bath and cover with at least an inch of water. Boil for ten minutes. Using jar tongs, carefully lift the jars out of the water bath and let them cool at room temperature. You will hear the lids seal when they make a popping noise as the domed lid is sucked down. Processed jam will last at least a year and makes a lovely gift. For small batches, you can make your jam and store it in the fridge as soon as it has cooled off. Berries contain protection magic as well as that of abundance. Folklore says vampires are afraid of blackberry vines.

Imbued with Love: Lavender Rosemary Infused Vodka

This clear alcoholic drink is also easily infused with the flavor of flowers, herbs, fruits and even vegetables. Try combinations such as the light and sweet floral taste of lavender and rosemary. Lavender brings calming and healing and rosemary dispels negative spirits. Both of these are love herbs. What could be better? You'll need the following:

- ⇛ A quart bottle of vodka
- ⇛ 2 sprigs of rosemary
- ⇛ 3 springs of lavender

⟫   Larger canning jar with sealable lid

After you have rinsed your herbs in cool water and gently patted them dry, put them in the one-quart (32 ounce) Mason or Bell jar. Pour in vodka, making sure to cover the herbs to the top, then seal tightly. Give it a vigorous shake and place the jar in your pantry or dark closet for five days, making sure to shake at least once a day. After the second day, take a spoon and taste the vodka. If the taste suits you before the full five days are up, go ahead and strain the herbs out using cheesecloth or a paper coffee filter, Set the herbs aside and let them dry. After the vodka is thoroughly strained of any herbs or residue, pour it into a bottle; label the bottle with the date and what herbs you used. Tie the dry herbs into a bundle with string and use their aroma when you next make a fire in the hearth. Their scentful smoke will imbue your home with coziness, calm, healing and love.

Auntie's Apple Brandy Spirits

Here is a delightfully easy recipe that will produce a flavorful homemade liqueur that smells as good as it tastes. If you are interested in making a hassle-free bottle of spirits, apples are a wonderful way to start. Start with these ingredients:

⟫   4 apples (sweet ones, not sour)

⟫   2 cups brandy

⟫   2 cups vodka

➥   1 quart clean and sterilized Mason jar

First, clean, core, and slice your apples. Place the slices in a Mason canning jar. Pour in the alcohol to cover, using equal parts brandy and vodka. Put the jar in a cool dark place in your pantry. Allow the infusion process to alchemize for a month or until it is to your taste. The combination of sweet apples and brandy gives a luscious fruit-forward flavor, with no need for sugar. After infusing, strain the apple slices out using a strainer to filter the liqueur. Pour the spirits into a pretty and sealable bottle and enjoy at your next pagan party.

Bonus tip: apples can really be used with any spirit so let your imagination run wild!

Astrological Herbology

You can also choose the herbs for your altar based on your sun or moon sign. Explore making tinctures, incenses, oils, potpourris, and other magical potions for your rituals using celestial correspondences. For example, if the new moon is in Aries when you are performing an attraction ritual, try using peppermint or fennel, two herbs sacred to the sign of the Ram. If you are creating a special altar for the time during which the sun is in the sign of Cancer, use incense oils, teas, and herbs corresponding to that astrological energy, including jasmine and lemon. These correspondences create a synthesis of energies that adds to the effectiveness of your magical work.

Lunar Almanac: Moon Signs of the Times

The astrological signs of the moon are of great significance. Each moon sign has special meanings set down through the centuries. Ancient and medieval folks paid strict attention to moon phases and moon signs for planting, harvesting, and canning and preserving stores for the long winter. Here is a guide to each sign with tried-and-true lore from olden days along with applications for today's rituals.

Aries is a barren and dry sign that is perfect for planting, weeding, haying, and harvesting. Moon in Aries is the optimum time for rituals pertaining to leadership, pioneering, ambition, and authority, as well as rebirth. Any healing regarding the face and head is more successful during Aries.

Taurus is an earthy and moist sign that is excellent for planting root crops like potatoes and peanuts. Love, money, and luxury are watchwords for the moon in Taurus. If you are buying real estate, moon in Taurus is an excellent time for that. Because the throat and neck are ruled by Taurus, this is a prime time both for singing and speaking.

Gemini is another dry sign that is a great time for mowing, cutting, and getting rid of plants or pests. Communication is improved during moon in Gemini. Healing of the arms and hands and pulmonary system is well advised during a Gemini moon.

Cancer is a fruitful watery sign conductive to planting; in fact, it is the most productive sign of all. Hearth and home are the focus now, and lunar rituals are well timed during moon in Cancer. Healing rituals for the stomach are best done at this time.

Leo is the driest and least fertile of all moon signs, good only for cutting and mowing. Leo moon is good for bravery, striking out in a new direction, like performing on stage or taking a position of authority. Matters of the heart and literal healing of that organ are auspicious and advisable now.

Virgo is both damp and barren, but is a great time for cultivation. Virgo moon is good for working hard and seeking employment, tending to all aspects of health and nutrition, and healing the nervous system and bowel.

Libra is both wet and fruitful and is wonderful for grains, vines, root crops, and flowers. Now is the time for artistic endeavors, romantic liaisons, and balancing your life. The lower back and kidneys can be restored to health during moon in Libra.

Scorpio is humid and bountiful and is good for all types of planting. Make your moves during moon in Scorpio. This sign is also conducive to plumbing the depths of the spirit and achieving psychic growth. Sex rituals are at their most potent during moon in Scorpio. Healing of the sensitive reproductive organs can happen during this moon time.

Sagittarius is another fire sign that is a poor time for planting and so is best spent harvesting and storing. Rites of passage and travel and rituals relating to higher truths and philosophical matters succeed during moon in Sagittarius. Sports and horses are also in the spotlight during this time. Healing for the legs can be undertaken during this time.

Capricorn is an earth sign that is also wet and is excellent for grafting, pruning, and planting trees and shrubs. Rituals relating to work, goals, and organizing can be commenced at this time. Political careers, dreams, and aspirations should be launched during moon in Capricorn. Skeletal wellness efforts are advisable during this cycle, as well.

Aquarius is an infertile and parched moon time that is best for harvesting, weeding, and dispelling pests. The Aquarian moon is appropriate for rites regarding personal freedom. Friendship, the intellect, and starting a new phase of life all come into play now. Rituals of a more radical nature are best during this sign. Shin and ankle health tend to go better now, too.

Pisces is fecund and fruitful and is good for all kinds of planting. It is remarkable for fruits of all kinds. The highly sensitive moon in Pisces is good for spells and charms for creativity, intuition, divination, dream work, and music. Care and healing for the feet are most favorable during this sign of moon in Pisces.

Blackberry Malt Vinegar Syrup

Blackberries are one of life's sweetest gifts, growing abundantly in the bramble along the rambling path. An extremely effective medicinal tonic can be made by soaking a quart of berries in a quart of malt vinegar for three days. Drain and strain the liquid into a pan. Simmer and stir in sugar, one pound to every two cups of tonic. Boil gently for five minutes and skim off any foam. Cool and pour into a sealable jar. This potion is so powerful, you can add a teaspoon into a cup of water and cure tummy aches, cramps, fevers, coughs, and colds. Best of all, blackberry vinegar is both a medicine and a highly prized dessert topping in the UK. Pour some over your apple pie and cream, and you will soon scurry off to pick blackberries all summer.

Fruitful Magic

While we often think of herbs and flowers as having special properties, it is much less commonly known that fruits also contain much magic you must try for yourself:

Apple

This beloved "one a day" fruit is associated with the goddess Pomona and contains the powers of healing, love and abundance. Samhain, the highest holiday of the Wheel of the Year, is also called the "Feast of Apples," and they are used on the Halloween altar during this festival. Cutting an apple in half and sharing the other half with your beloved is a traditional way to make a wish that the two of you will stay happy together for as long as apple trees grow.

Apricot

This juicy treasure is associated with Venus and the power of love, and it is believed that drinking the nectar will make you more appealing romantically. The juice of the apricot is used in rituals and love potions. Truly a food of the goddess!

Avocado

The lusciousness of the avocado fruit is not just delicious, it also brings forth beauty and lustfulness.

Banana

A bunch of bananas packs a magical punch with powers of abundance and fertility for both men and women. Anyone who gets married beneath a banana tree bower will have a lucky marriage. One caveat: never cut a banana open, only break it apart. Otherwise, you'll bring bad luck to your household.

Blackberry

Blackberries are the medicine that pops up anywhere, offering a delightful snack and serious healing, love, and abundance. Both the vine and the berries can be used for money-bringing spells. Thorny blackberry vines are wonderful as protective wreaths for your home, and the plant's vine and berry can be used for prosperity and money spells.

Blueberry

These berries are almost like an evil eye charm made of fruit, since they offer great protection. You can tuck a few of them under the mat at the threshold of your front door to ward off bad energy and evil if you feel someone is attempting to do you harm with hexes or sending bad energy your way,

Cherry

Beloved for their bright red color and taste, cherries are associated with romance as well as powers of divination. Useful in love spells, the Japanese believe tying a strand of hair from your head onto the blossom of a cherry tree will bring a lover to you.

Figs

Figs hold a place in our culture from the story of Adam and Eve in the Garden of Eden. Unsurprisingly, they are associated with sexuality and fecundity. If eaten ripe off the tree, this fruit will aid in conception and helps men with issues of impotence. A fig tree, if grown outside the bedroom, will bring deeply restful sleep and prophetic dreams. Outside your kitchen, a fig tree will ensure there will always be plenty of food for your family. Anywhere a fig tree grows it will bring luck and safety. A folk charm claims that gifting someone a fig grown by your own hand binds them to you. Wield your figs wisely.

Grapes

Planting grapevines grants abilities for money magic as well as with gardening and farming: the ancient Romans painted pictures of grapes on the garden walls to ensure good harvest and fertility for women. For mental focus, eat some grapes; magical spell workings for money are abetted greatly by placing a bowl of grapes on the altar.

Lemon

This beloved member of the citrus family confers the rare power of longevity as well as those of faithful friendship, purification, love, and luck. The juice from a lemon mixed with water can be used to consecrate magical tools and items during the full moon. Dried lemon flowers and peel can also be used in love potions and sachets. Bake a lemon pie for the object of your desire, and he or she will remain faithful to you for all time. Imbibing lemon leaf tea stirs lust.

Orange

In keeping with the joyful color of this fruit, oranges are a fruit of happiness in love and marriage. Dried blossoms added to a hot bath make you more beautiful. A spritz of orange juice will add to the potency of any love potion, especially if freshly squeezed. Orange sachets, pomanders, and other gifts with this fruit offer the recipient utter felicity; thus, it is an ideal gift for newlyweds.

Peach

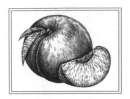 It might seem obvious, but eating peaches encourages love. They also enhance wisdom. An amulet made with the pit can ward off evil. A fallen branch from a peach tree can make an excellent magic wand, while a piece of the tree's wood carried in your pocket is an excellent talisman for a long life.

Pear

It is believed this uniquely shaped fruit brings prosperity and a long life. Somewhat similarly to peaches, the pear correlates with powers of lust and love. By sharing them with a partner, pears can be used to induce sexual arousal; pears cooked in wine or with a little rum or brandy make for an irresistible dessert with a little whipped cream. Pear wood is also very good for magical wands.

Pineapple

While renowned as the symbol of hospitality, pineapple represents neighborliness, abundance, and chastity. Dried pineapple in a sachet added to bath water will bring great luck. The juice hinders lust when drunken, and its dried peel is great in money spells and mixtures.

Plum

Plums are for protection and add sweetness to romantic love. A fallen (not cut) branch from a plum tree over the door keeps out negative energy and wards off evil.

Pomegranate

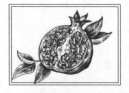 Here we have powers of divination, making wishes come true, and engendering wealth. Eating the seeds can increase fruitfulness in childbearing; you can also carry the rind in a pocket sachet. Always make a wish before eating the fruit, for your wish will come true.

Raspberry

This sweet berry has tremendous powers for true love and safety in your home. Hang the vines at all of a house's doors when a person in the house has died so that the spirit won't enter the home again. The leaves are carried by pregnant woman to help with the pains of childbirth and pregnancy itself. Raspberries often served to induce love. Strawberry leaves also help with childbirth and the leaves are also carried for luck.

Tomato

Reminder that like the "alligator pear" or avocado, the tomato is a fruit! An easy money spell is to place a fresh-off-the-vine tomato on the mantle every few days to bring prosperity. Eating tomatoes inspires love. They are excellent to plant in your garden as an aid to ward off pests of all kinds!

House Sweet Home Orchard Potpourri

Even if you don't have a have a citrus orchard out back, you can still make your own home-freshening mix of potpourri. Even better, you can make lemonade, limeade, or orange juice, then slice up the remainder of the fruit. Lay the rind and slices on a big sheet pan and let them dry. Add dried rose petals, bunches of lavender and rosemary, or dried sprigs of mint for a wonderfully fresh scent. Tuck into muslin bags and tie up with a pretty and colorful ribbon and you have a lovely all-occasion gift for housewarmings and holidays, one that is truly a blessing for any home.

Lemon Aid: Healthful Lemon Curd

We all know the adage that starts out, "when life gives you lemons," but we would update this classic with the suggestion to make lemon curd! With only four ingredients, it is not a complex chore but a delightful way to take your bounty of citrus and create a sweet and creamy joy-filled treat for you and your loved ones to enjoy for many months to come. What you'll need:

- ➤➤ 8 whole lemons (Meyer lemons are ideal, but any and all lemons will do)
- ➤➤ 2½ cups white sugar, granulated
- ➤➤ 2 cups fresh, unsalted butter
- ➤➤ 8 whole eggs, beaten

Have at the ready: eight clean glass jars previously sterilized in hot water; half-pint Mason jars preferred.

Grate the zest of the lemons into a medium-sized saucepan. Squeeze the juice from the lemons into a bowl, go for every drop! You should have around 1½ cups of juice. Add the lemon juice to the saucepan along with the sugar. Cut butter into small pieces and add to the pan gradually.

Place your saucepan on a burner over low heat and stir until the butter melts and the sugar dissolves. Strain the beaten eggs through a fine-mesh sieve into the pan with the lemon mixture. Cook on a medium heat for ten to fifteen minutes, stirring frequently. As it heats up, the mixture will begin to thicken and take on a creamy consistency. When it coats the back of a spoon, you are well on your way to lemon curd!

When the lemon sauce is thick, remove the pan from the heat. Fill hot sterilized jars with the lemon curd to within ⅛ inch of rims. Wipe the rims clean, then top the jars with hot lids. Screw down the bands securing the lids onto the jars until finger tight. Process jars in a hot water bath for ten minutes. Remove jars and stand them upright on a clean towel, away from drafts. Let jars sit undisturbed for twelve hours. Check for proper seals. Label the jars and store in a cool, dry place for up to a year.

Longevity Elixir: Homemade Pear Potion

Pears have long been prized in Asia as a lucky fruit that also nourishes a long and prosperous life. The great magical teacher Scott Cunningham advocated for their use in love spells. This pear liqueur is a special brew indeed. You will need this to make it:

- ⇛ 3 large ripe pears
- ⇛ 2 pods of cardamom
- ⇛ Lemon peel of half a lemon
- ⇛ Vodka, 1 quart
- ⇛ 1 clean and sterilized 1-quart Mason jar with lid (preferably dark-colored glass)

Start by crushing the cardamom pods, then set aside. Peel the pears and cut into thin slices. Gently place the pear slices into the jar. Put the crushed cardamom and lemon peel on top of the pears. Cover all with the vodka. Close the jar and tighten the lid, then gently shake twice. Store the jar full of pears in a dark, cool cupboard for ten days. After the ten days, remove the jar from the cupboard. Pour the contents of the jar into a mixing bowl and mash thoroughly using the back of a fork. Strain the mixture into another bowl, using a colander that has been lined with a coffee filter or cheesecloth. Repeat this process twice, then pour the pear liqueur into the Mason jar. (The strained-out pear slices can be consumed or used in cookery, but remember that they may be quite potent!) If you are feeling fancy, you can store your pear liqueur in a pretty bottle. Live long and prosper!

DIY Detoxing

Herbal Decoctions

To make a tea from the root, bark, or stems of plants, you will need to make a decoction; add approximately two tablespoons of the herb to one cup of water and gently simmer covered on a very low flame for half an hour.

Dandy Sassafras Ginger Detox

When I was little and living on the family farm, I accompanied my dad to the woods looking for sassafras roots to make tea. I loved the taste; it was delightful and gave me more energy. After apprenticing with my part-Cherokee dad for a few years, he allowed me to go out alone to gather the source of my dearly beloved beverage. Years later, I discovered sassafras was highly prized by Native Americans who used it for medicine and were extremely knowledgeable about combining herbs to amplify their power.

This morning medicinal is inspired by a shamanic Native healing recipe using sassafras, dandelion root, and wild ginger root. For a wonderfully medicinal decoction, take a half cup of each and boil them in spring water. After simmering for twelve minutes, stir in honey and enjoy. It is pleasantly surprising how good the detox tastes and even more amazing how the herbs combine to eliminate toxins from the body, chiefly the kidney and liver. During the holidays or at pagan feast times, we all may tend to imbibe and enjoy rich foods, good wine, and sugary desserts. This purifying herbal blend will cleanse the organs that cleanse your body, thus aiding wellness. This detox should be used seasonally and is not intended for daily use due to its great power.

Decoctions 101

Infusion as a method doesn't work well with roots, barks, and herbs with tough stems and seeds. Decocting is bringing the pot nearly to a boil and then reducing by simmering slowly to produce the most concentrated liquid, which is excellent in medicines. Use a well-cleaned coffee grinder for roots and small pieces of bark and stems to make quick work of these. I recommend the decoction method for the roots of willow, sarsaparilla, wild cherry, yohimbe, yucca, licorice, parsley, dandelion, angelica, and cohosh.

Healing Secrets of the Ancients

Oxymel is a very old-fashioned tonic that dates back to ancient times but has fallen out of fashion. It remains a favorite used by herbal healers and it is made of two seemingly opposing ingredients—honey and vinegar. Herbs can be added to great effect, and when you see honey menthol cough drops on the pharmacy shelf, note their origin in traditions that began over two thousand years ago. Oxymels are supremely effective for respiratory issues. The recipe is simplicity itself: equal parts honey and vinegar poured over herbs in a canning jar. Store in a dark cupboard and give the sealed jar a good shake every day. After two weeks, strain out the herbs with cheesecloth and store your oxymel in the fridge.

Recommended oxymel herbs: oregano, elder flower, sage, balm, mint, lemon peel, thyme, lavender, rose petals, hyssop, and fennel.

Craft Your Own Cough Drops: Candied Herbs

- ⟫ 1 cup vodka
- ⟫ 1 cup simple syrup
- ⟫ 1 cup honey
- ⟫ 2 cups dried herb (of your choice)
- ⟫ 1 large sheet waxed paper

One of the byproducts of making herbal honeys, liqueurs, and oxymel is the candied herbs, which can also be made especially for snacks and for use in sweetcakes and cookies. To make a batch, stir the liquids together in a big pot and heat slowly, stirring every few minutes. Upon reaching boiling point, add the herbs until well mixed. Turn the heat down and slowly simmer until the liquid is very thick and sticky. Spoon the herbs out and place on wax paper to crystallize. Good herbs for this are hyssop, ginger root, lavender, lemon balm, fennel seed, mint, angelica stems, and thyme as well as small slivers of orange, lime, and lemon. The gift of homemade candy is a marvelous way to signal a crush.

CHAPTER SEVEN

Essential Oils and Aromatherapy: Harness Healing Power

. . . .

Essential oils have been used medicinally for centuries. They are extracted from flowers, grasses, shrubs, herbs, and trees. If you are skeptical about the efficacy of essential oils, you'll at least find it reassuring to know that the oils enter and exit the human body without leaving any toxins behind. The best ways to use essential oils are externally, absorbed through the skin, or through steam inhalation. However, oral applications are indicated for some remedies.

How to Use Essential Oils

Most of the home remedies I personally prefer are either essential oil massage treatments or essential oils diffused into the bath or air. The best base oils for essential oils are cold-pressed vegetable and seed or nut oils. The most affordable are sunflower, safflower, corn, and grapeseed. Add essential oils to base oil at a ratio of one drop per five milliliters. Twenty drops of an essential oil come out to approximately one milliliter, so add twenty drops to a hundred milliliters of base oil.

A few drops of an essential oil from a dropper in the bath is sufficient for therapeutic use, and a few drops in water in a diffuser will fill a room with healing molecules. A drop on a cotton ball wiped on a light bulb or on a radiator will also gently diffuse the oil into the air. Here's another helpful tip: try a few drops in a small bowl of very hot water. Shut the doors and windows, and the essence will permeate a room in five minutes. This is a particularly easy way to create a nice ambience in a room with soothingly scented air.

My sister suffers from osteoarthritis in her shoulder. She takes baths with synergistic blends of fourteen essential oils: fennel, cypress, juniper, cedarwood, sandalwood, petitgrain, pine, ginger, lavender, rosemary, black pepper, birch, nutmeg, and marjoram. These, combined with sea salt and Epsom salts, have turned her into a true believer in the amazing therapeutic effects of essential oils!

There are hundreds of essential oils used by herbalists, but for general therapeutic use in the home, these are my recommendations as far as what you need to have at the ready.

Lavender Oil

If I could only have one essential oil, I would choose lavender because it is so versatile. It is a natural antibiotic, antiseptic, sedative, antidepressant, topical treatment for scalds and burns, and a good detoxifier; it prevents scarring and promotes healing, and its lovely scent has a calming effect that is widely used in aromatherapy.

Tea Tree Oil

Used by aborigines in Australia for centuries, tea tree oil is a powerful antibacterial, antifungal, and antiseptic. It has a fresh camphor smell and is used to treat athlete's foot, sunburn, candida, dandruff, pimples, gum disease, and other infections. Be careful not to use it *undiluted* without careful sensitivity testing first, as it is potently aromatic! It can make a useful addition to formulations ranging from shampoo to mouthwash to herbal hand sanitizer and liquid soap.

Peppermint Oil

A wonderful therapeutic for digestive, respiratory, and circulatory complaints, peppermint oil is used to treat indigestion, irritable bowel syndrome, flatulence, halitosis, catarrh, varicose veins, headaches, skin irritations, and rheumatism. It also works as a deterrent for infestations of mice, fleas, and ants. It is not surprising that peppermint oil is regarded as the world's oldest medicine. Paradoxically, peppermint is useful to support either alertness or relaxation as it will nourish whatever you need in terms of balancing your day-to-day energy.

Eucalyptus Oil

In eucalyptus oil, we have an all-purpose antiviral, antibiotic, diuretic, analgesic, and antiseptic. It can be therapeutic for coughs, colds, respiratory stimulation, and insect bites. If you start to feel cold symptoms, use five drops of eucalyptus oil in a hot bath or in a bowl prepared with boiling water for a head steam.

Thyme Oil

Thyme is an "old-time" antiviral, antibiotic, antiseptic, and diuretic curative; it was highly valued and widely used by the ancient Egyptians, Greeks, and Romans for fatigue, coughs, warts, rheumatism, neuralgia, and acne. Thyme oil works very well mixed with base oil for massage.

Rosemary Oil

Sweet-smelling rosemary oil is a great antiseptic to use for flu and coughs, as well as helpful with headaches, depression, muscular stress, arthritis, rheumatism, fatigue, and forgetfulness. Rosemary oil is stimulating and will perk you up if you do a head steam with it or put a couple of drops in the bath.

Aromatherapeutic Quality Control

Essential oils are highly concentrated extracts of flowers, herbs, root, or resins, sometimes diluted in a neutral base oil. Try to ensure you are using natural oils instead of manufactured, chemical-filled perfume oil; the synthetics lack any real energy. Also, approach oils with caution and don't get them in your eyes. Clean cotton gloves are a good idea to keep in your kitchen for handling sensitive materials. You can avoid any mess and protect your magical tools by using oil droppers. While you are learning and studying, find a trusted herbalist or the wise sage at your local metaphysical shop; usually their years of experience offer much in the way of useful knowledge you can use to your advantage. I have included as much as I can in this at-a-glance guide to oils:

These essential oils are excellent choices for anointing lamps as well as yourself:

- ⇛ **Cinnamon** is energetic, spicy, and warm. It stimulates the mind as well as the body.

- ⇛ **Ginger** is vigorous and revitalizing and heightens desire and comfort.

- ⇛ **Jasmine** sparks sensuality and inspires feelings of positivity, confidence, and pure bliss.

- ⇛ **Lavender** is soothing, calming, nurturing, and relaxing.

- ⇛ **Orange** is a light, citrusy oil that restores balance and lifts moods while enhancing playful emotions.

- **Rose** brings youthfulness, enhances self-esteem, aids circulation, and relieves tension.

- **Sandalwood** is a woody aroma that relieves tension and relaxes tense muscles.

- **Ylang-ylang**'s sweet floral aroma is used as an aphrodisiac; it is relaxing and reduces worry and anxiety.

Carrier Oils

A carrier oil is a vegetable oil that is used to dilute essential oils without diminishing the effect of the essence. It ensures that essential oils used topically are comfortable on the skin. Each essence carries specific vibrations that hold much curative power. These base oils support other ingredients including essential oils and can also be agents for healing in themselves.

Apricot kernel oil, with its warmth and resilience, is especially good for women. Apricot protects love and nurtures women at every age and stage of life.

 Avocado is thick, dense, and earthy, a powerful element in any love potion. It also is excellent for drawing forth money and is helpful in business and financial matters.

Borage oil brings a connection with the higher mind, as well as courage, a sense of honor, and the ability to cope with whatever life sends your way. It is said to encourage truth and resolution in legal and relationship problems. If you feel you are being deceived, turn to borage.

Evening primrose oil abets clairvoyance and paranormal gifts. It will help you to see clearly.

Grapeseed oil is regarded by some as the "food of the gods" because of the way it augments spiritual growth. This should be one of the oils that you turn to for anointing yourself or any statuary of gods and goddess before rituals.

Jojoba oil absorbs extremely well into the skin, bearing anything with which it is mixed along with it. It is also a remarkable anointing oil. It should be used in recipes that help to deal with depression and support perseverance in hardship.

 Olive oil was named "liquid gold" by the ancient Greek poet Homer, and rightly so: it is about vitality, money, success, and joyfulness.

Sunflower oil, permeated with the energy of our sun, is powerful and life-giving. Use it when you desire rapid growth and amplification of positive energy.

Sweet almond is a gentle, all-purpose oil ready to increase the energy of other ingredients.

Simple Remedies for Common Maladies

Valerie Worwood's *The Fragrant Pharmacy* is one of my bibles for learning about essential oils. Since I discovered essential oils and aromatherapy, I've been developing my own recipes. Often, I'll amend a recipe to just one or two oils that I have on hand.

Itchy Skin and Feet

Either use a few drops of undiluted tea tree oil on the affected area, or massage with a drop of tea tree oil in a teaspoon of vegetable oil if there are issues with sensitive skin.

Cuts

Stanch an open wound with lavender oil on a cotton ball. Bandage a cut with a drop of lavender oil on the gauze, changing the dressing morning and night, and leave the wound uncovered as much as possible from the third day onward.

Bruises

Add two drops of lavender oil and two drops of rosemary oil to a bowl of hot water and the same to a bowl of cold water. Alternately apply to the bruised area a washcloth soaked in the hot infusion and one soaked in the cold infusion.

Burns

Leave the area where the burn is under running cold water for fifteen minutes, then apply two drops of neat (undiluted) lavender oil to the burn. Cover the area with a gauze compress soaked in cold water and three drops of lavender oil.

Boils

Add three drops of lavender oil and three drops of tea tree oil to a small bowl of hot water and bathe the area twice a day.

Chest Coughs

Prepare a bowl of boiling water for steam inhalation with one drop of rosemary, two drops of peppermint, and one drop of eucalyptus, draping a towel over your head to create a tent for the steam. Make massage oil for chest and back with one drop of lavender, three drops of rosemary, four drops of eucalyptus, and one drop of thyme in a level tablespoon of a vegetable base oil.

Dry Hacking Cough

Make a honey and lemon hot toddy, adding one drop of eucalyptus essential oil. Massage chest and back with two drops each of eucalyptus and thyme in a level tablespoon of a vegetable base oil. For a head steam, add either two drops of lavender or two drops of eucalyptus to the hot water.

Cold Sores

Apply tea tree oil directly to the sore morning and night.

Colds

Make a bowl of hot water for inhalation with one drop each of thyme, lavender, and eucalyptus oils. For a hot bath, add two drops each of thyme, lavender, and tea tree oil. Soak in the bath, relaxing your muscles and breathing deeply.

Upset Stomach

Always be sure to drink a lot of water when you are afflicted with a digestive malady, being careful not to chug it. If the cause is related to what food you ate, make a drink with a teaspoon of honey and a drop of peppermint oil in warm water. If you think you have a virus or nervous tummy, make a drink with warm water, a teaspoon of honey, and a drop of eucalyptus oil.

Headache

For a general headache, massage temples with a drop of either lavender or peppermint oil, or both together. You can also use rosemary or clove oil, but you will need to experiment, as some essentials will work better for you than others. If the headache is related to an upset tummy, mix a drop of peppermint oil with a teaspoon of honey dissolved in a cup of warm water and sip slowly.

Toothache

Place one drop of clove oil on a cotton swab and apply directly to the tooth and the surrounding gum. If you have a decayed tooth waiting to be treated, apply a paste made of goldenseal powder and water to the affected area. It tastes bitter but will prevent an infection from setting in until you can see a dentist.

Aromatherapeutic Massage Oils

Massage oils can be made in minutes if you have the ingredients on hand; head to your nearest health food store and get the raw ingredients. I am one lucky lady to have a soap and candle store in my neighborhood, Juniper Tree in Berkeley, California. I am found there twice a month picking up what I need, from candle wicks to essential and base oils and plain bath salts for my custom creations. Record your experiments with various oils in a journal. After several moons, note which had the best results for you and which you preferred. For example, if you received a proposal of marriage after a Very Vanilla soaking session, I'd say that works for you!

Mystical Meanings of Essential Oils

Astral Projection: jasmine, benzoin, cinnamon, sandalwood

Courage: geranium, black pepper, frankincense

Dispelling Negative Energy and Spirits: basil, clove, copal, frankincense, juniper, myrrh, pine, peppermint, rosemary, Solomon's seal, yarrow, vervain

Divination: camphor, orange, clove

Enchantment: ginger, tangerine, amber, apple

Healing: bay laurel, cedarwood, cinnamon, coriander, eucalyptus, juniper, lime, rose, sandalwood, spearmint

Joy: lavender, neroli, bergamot, vanilla

Love: apricot, basil, chamomile, clove, copal, coriander, rose, geranium, jasmine, lemon, lime, neroli, rosemary, ylang-ylang

Luck: orange, nutmeg, rose, vervain

Peace: lavender, chamomile

Prosperity: basil, clove, ginger, cinnamon, nutmeg, orange, oak, moss, patchouli, peppermint, pine, aloe

Protection: bay laurel, anise, black pepper, cedar, clove, cypress, copal, eucalyptus, frankincense, rose geranium, lime, myrrh, lavender, juniper, sandalwood, vetiver

Sexuality: Cardamom, lemongrass, amber, rose, clove, olive, patchouli

Breathe Easy: Keep Colds at Bay

Banish colds and coughs or keep them at bay with this sweet-smelling breath enhancer. In a blue bottle, shake the following essential oils:

- ⫸ 10 drops rosemary
- ⫸ 10 drops tea tree
- ⫸ 10 drops eucalyptus
- ⫸ 10 drops lavender
- ⫸ One teaspoon sea salt

Hold the open container in both hands under your nose and breathe deeply three times.

You can administer this respiratory booster by adding four drops either to the water of a vaporizer or diffuser or to a cotton ball tucked into your pillowcase. Six drops poured into the running water of a hot bath will ease breathing immediately

Soothing Sandalwood Meditation

Sandalwood, lavender, and clary sage create a deeply relaxing blend with a warm and soothing scent. Here is what you need:

- ⫸ 6 tablespoons almond oil
- ⫸ 2 tablespoons jojoba oil

- 20 drops sandalwood essential oil

- 15 drops lavender essential oil

- 5 drops clary sage essential oil

Mix oils together in a tightly capped blue, dark green, or brown bottle. Shake well and pour a bit into the palm of your hand to warm before using. Rub it lightly onto your shoulder and neck as well as your temples and wrists. Sit comfortably and breathe deeply with your eyes closed. Chant aloud:

> *Remove from me all worry.*
> *Remove all stress in a hurry.*
> *No more will I lack sleep.*
> *No more will I weep.*
> *Tranquility and calm, come to me now.*

Scent of Serenity Mist

My aunt Edith, who introduced me to the wonders of gardening, had a linen closet that always smelled sweetly of lavender. I remember breathing in the smell and immediately feeling comforted. Sleeping on crisp, clean, herb-scented sheets always made for the soundest sleep and delicious dreams. (Little did I know at the time, lavender is also a moth repellent and an adaptogen, adjusting to satisfy your own energy needs.) Here is a potion for dreamers:

- 4 drops lavender oil

- 3 drops chamomile oil

- 3 drops orange oil

- 4 ounces distilled spring water

Shake the oils and water in a colored glass spray bottle or mister.

Fifteen minutes before you retire, spray your bed linens, bath towel, pillow, and all around your room. You may want to keep a dream journal by your bed to record what happens during the night.

Aromatherapy for Anxiety: The Scent of Serenity

Rose essential oil is extracted from the flower's petals and has an exquisite perfume. Rose is also highly prized for how it relaxes and stimulates the senses and memory.

Lavender is one of the most beloved of all aromatherapy oils, not just for its singular scent; it has been proven to relieve tension by the reaction of the limbic system in the brain that controls our emotions.

Jasmine essential oil has an arresting floral scent which can cause an increased sense of well-being. Jasmine calms the nervous system without causing sleepiness.

Vetiver oil is derived from the vetiver plant, a grassy native of India. It has a sweet, earthy scent and is used to attain a meditative state and is a marvelous anti-anxiety remedy as well.

Basil essential oil comes from the same herb that you use in cooking. In aromatherapy, it's used to help calm the mind and alleviate stress.

Clary Sage is a woody essential oil that is valued for its antidepressant qualities. It has been proven to reduce the body's production of the hormone cortisol, known as the "stress hormone."

Bergamot comes from bergamot oranges and has a revitalizing citrusy scent. Bergamot is beloved for how it can uplift and improve mood.

Ylang-Ylang is highly floral and a great relaxant. It is also proven in scientific tests to lower tension, reduce blood pressure, and even out the heart rate.

Chamomile is pretty well-known for its relaxing and sedating properties and appealing scent; it can help overcome sleep disruptions and bring about a good, deep rest.

Frankincense oil is made from a tree resin and has been cherished for its sweetly musky yet purifying aroma, which is used to create a meditative state and ease anxiety.

Lemon Balm has a bracing and uplifting scent which is very soothing and restorative; it can also be a sleep aid.

Valerian: an herb that has been used since ancient times to promote sleep and calm nerves. It has a tranquilizing and sedative effect on the body.

Patchouli also has a musky woodsy scent and is used in ayurvedic medicine to relieve anxiety, stress, and depression.

Power Potpourri

Simmer this mixture on your stove whenever you feel the need to infuse your space with protection or do an energetic turnaround from negative to positive. When a bad day at work, a family squabble, or an unfortunate incident in your neighborhood happens, instead of just muddling along, you can do something about it, and your creating positive energy will help you and your loved ones as well as your neighbors. This Power Potpourri will also safeguard your home from outside influences that can be disruptive. Set your intention and gather these herbs together:

- ¼ cup rosemary
- 4 bay laurel leaves
- ⅛ cup sage
- 1 teaspoon juniper berries

Mix the herbs together by hand. While you are stirring, close your eyes and visualize your home protected by a boundary of glowing white light. Imagine the light runs through you to the herbs in your hand and charges them with the energy of safety, sanctity, and protection. Add the herbs to slowly simmering water and breathe in the newly charged air.

Sacred Self-Care Pampering Potion

This relaxation remedy is an excellent way to create personal space after a hectic week. In a small pottery bowl or vial, mix together the following essential oils with a small amount of base oil:

- ➤➤ 2 drops cedar oil
- ➤➤ 2 drops sandalwood
- ➤➤ 2 drops ylang-ylang
- ➤➤ 2 drops lavender

Add this mixture to a mild carrier oil (olive or almond, for example) and rub one drop on each pulse point: on both wrists, behind your ear lobes, on the base of your neck, and behind your knees. As the oil surround you with its warm scent, you will be filled with a quiet strength.

Blissful Balm

With this blissful combination of oils, you can summon the spirit of love and harmony any day of the year. Amber, rose, and sandalwood create a sensual scent that lingers on your skin for hours.

- ➤➤ 6 tablespoons almond oil
- ➤➤ 2 tablespoons jojoba oil
- ➤➤ 25 drops sandalwood essential oil

⤜   3 drops rose essential oil

⤜   5 drops amber essential oil

Mix oils together in a dark blue, brown, or dark green bottle, cap it tightly, and shake well. You now have an aphrodisiac in a bottle; use it on your skin whenever you wish to summon love.

Flower and herb-based aromatherapy essences can also be used in diffusers to infuse the air with the desired fragrance. Many of the most sensual essential oils combine well together: Try a combination of amber and apple, or ylang-ylang and sandalwood, clary sage and rose, and sweet almond and neroli. If you're using a candle diffuser, rose or orange blossom water is an aromatic and romantic alternative to using plain water in the diffuser cup.

Additional romantic touches include fresh flowers, which can be used in creative ways. In Indonesia, lily and orange blossom flowers are scattered on a newlywed couple's bed. You can also make a trail of blossoms for your lover to follow; scatter rose petals on your bed or surround your bed with a garland of flowers. Plenty of pillows for lounging, sensuous silk or chenille throws for staying cozy, and your favorite mood-setting music all help cast a spell of romance.

Aphrodisiac essential oils include clary sage, jasmine, neroli, patchouli, rose, sandalwood, vanilla, vetiver, and ylang-ylang.

Lavender and Mint Energy Cleanser: Clearing Vibrational Clutter

In order to do any ritual work, you must first clear the clutter that can create blocks. Banish the old, bad energy from your house by following this spell. Make your energy-clearing tea by bringing four cups of water to a full rolling boil; remove from heat and add in four sprigs of fresh lavender and four sprigs of fresh mint. If it is winter and there is no access to fresh herbs, one tablespoon each of dried lavender and dried mint will do nicely. Steep the herbal tea covered for at least four minutes or as long as ten minutes if there is a lot of energetic clutter. Once it cools, dip your finger in the tea and sprinkle it throughout your home. If you feel the need to clear out any remaining clouds of psychic clutter, add diluted lavender mint tea water to your cleanser when you wash floors or surfaces. The scent of calm and clarity will lift the spirits of all who enter your space.

Herbal Clutter Busters

Sweetgrass: Native Americans have burned braided sheaves of sweetgrass for centuries. It is so scentful, it can even be wafted around as a wand to clear energy without lighting it. Native folks also brew a tea from it to use as an astringent body and hair rinse; you can do this by steeping a tablespoon of the dried chopped sweetgrass for five minutes in a standard teapot or two cups of boiling water. It is also used as an adornment either woven into braids or as a crown. They go by the philosophy that "strong hair means a strong mind." This power herb cleanses both body, soul, and your home, but its highest use is for rituals when you burn it to call forth the ancestors and send away anything unwanted.

Copal: Mexican and South American tribal healers and modern shamans gather this tree resin to employ as ceremonial incense throughout the year. You can still smell the sweetly pungent smoke of copal on the Day of the Dead as it helps us connect with our ancestors and loved ones who passed to the other side. While burning it is part of the ritual, it is also believed by shamans and healers to help tap into the spiritual realm. Copal also has the power to bring about total relaxation. As with other resins, burn it on a small disc of incense charcoal, which can be acquired at your local spiritual supply shop or botanica.

Palo Santo: This dried wood plays an important role in South American cultures, where it is burned to clear spaces of bad energy. It also activates a higher power in those who use it. Smelling the scent of Palo Santo clears out psychic clutter and purifies both you and your environment. It is said it literally burns away negative thoughts in your mind, a deeply powerful experience.

The Scent of Happiness

The minute you walk into someone's home, you can almost immediately tell how happy a household it is. Much of that is determined by the smell. A home with the fragrance of sugar cookies or a freshly baked pumpkin pie is one you may well want to visit often. Similarly, a space redolent of the bouquet of lilies or tea roses is one where the residents take care to make their home beautiful to both the eye and the other senses. There are lots of small things we can do in regard to "energy maintenance" for our home. To sweeten any mood, this recipe works wonders on you or anyone in your environment who might need a lift. Combine the following essential oils:

- 〽 2 drops neroli
- 〽 4 drops bergamot
- 〽 4 drops lavender
- 〽 2 drops rosemary

Add the mixture to a quart of distilled or fresh spring water and spray the air for an easy home makeover!

CHAPTER EIGHT

Practices to Accompany Your Herbal Cures

. . . .

Creating a sacred healing space will help safeguard your physical health and that of your loved ones. This table or workspace will be charged with your personal power. To ensure healthful beginnings, take two green candles and place them in green glass holders or votive glasses and position them in the two farthest corners. Place an incense burner in the center between the two candles and light some incense. Sandalwood, cinnamon, camphor, and frankincense are all powerful purification incenses. Burn one or all of these purification essences to consecrate the space—whatever represents healing energy to you. You may perhaps choose a candleholder carved from a chunk of amethyst crystal, which contains healing properties; an abalone shell with the iridescent magic of the oceans; a sweet-smelling bundle of sage; a small citrus plant bursting with the restorative power of vitamins; or a bowl of curative salts from the sea.

These symbolic items, and any others that you select, will energize your sacred space with the magic that lives inside you.

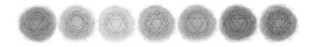

Chakra Tonics: Laying on of Stones

This healing practice is distilled from the study of chakras. Here are just a few examples of how to apply stones directly upon your body or that of anyone else who needs healing. By working with your chakras, you can become much more in touch with your body and soul.

The root chakra is at the base of your spine and is associated with passion, survival, security, and the color red. Above it is the sacral chakra in the lower abdominal region, which corresponds to such physical urges as hunger and sexuality; the color is orange. The solar plexus chakra is yellow and is associated with personal power. The heart chakra is green and symbolizes harmony, creativity, health, abundance, and nature. It is the energy center where the soul color of yellow and the spiritual color of blue combine. The throat chakra is blue and is considered the center of communication. The third eye chakra is located in the center of your forehead; it is associated with intuition and the color indigo. The crown chakra at the very top of your head is your connection to the universe and is violet in color.

The first step for anyone undertaking crystal healing is to lie down, relax, and get very comfortable. Empty everything else from your mind.

Lapis lazuli and its fellow blue gemstone aquamarine can be laid upon the throat chakra to release any blockage therein. This greatly aids in self-expression and is wonderful for professional speakers as well as performers such as actors and singers. Turquoise laid on the face—cheeks, forehead, and chin—is a calming agent that significantly reduces tension. Azurite on the brow opens the third eye and deepens wisdom; this can balance the energy of the head and allow more light into the third eye.

Malachite, a green heart stone, when placed near the heart and along the center of the abdomen will create a sense of harmony and facilitate letting go of pain, suffering, and old childhood wounds.

The rainbow is a simple and effective method for total body wellness. Choose from this list of stones, making sure you have one of each color of the rainbow—violet, indigo, blue, green, yellow, orange, and red—plus one white stone and one black stone for completion. Then, simply lay the stones on their corresponding chakra centers. I've included a list of crystal and body affinities in case there is any specific area you want to focus on:

Root Chakra

- jasper for the shins and for the skin
- garnet for the blood
- purple fluorite for the bone marrow
- jadeite for the knees
- chrysoprase for the prostate

Sacral Chakra

- moonstone for the womb area
- carnelian for the liver
- celestite for the intestines
- orange calcite for the bladder
- hematite for the liver and circulatory system

Solar Plexus Chakra

- chrysocolla for the pancreas
- fire agate for the stomach
- danburite for the muscles
- chalcedony for the spleen
- fire agate for the stomach

Heart Chakra

- rose quartz for the heart
- chrysolite for the appendix
- blue tourmaline for the thymus
- dioptase for the lungs

- ❥ moldavite for the hands
- ❥ moss agate for circulation and immune boosting

Throat Chakra

- ❥ amber for the thyroid
- ❥ lapis lazuli for the throat
- ❥ fluorite for the teeth
- ❥ calcite for the skeletal system

Third Eye Chakra

- ❥ benitoite for the pituitary
- ❥ beryl for the eyes
- ❥ calcite for the skeletal system
- ❥ dendrite agate for the nervous system

Crown Chakra

- ❥ citrine protects the aura
- ❥ Herkimer diamond for centered awareness
- ❥ coral calms and soothes nerves
- ❥ fluorite for coordination and balance
- ❥ amethyst for sobriety

Rite Before Surgery

There are certain occasions in life that, although extremely difficult, offer enormous opportunities for learning. One of these occasions is illness. I am a breast cancer survivor and have experienced several surgeries and lengthy recoveries. I will be forever grateful for my beloved friends who came together to support me and offer healing and love before the surgeries. My doctors were amazed at how well I healed; one female surgeon told me I was healing faster than any patient she had ever worked with before. I told her I believed it was because of the healing ritual we had performed. She was fascinated and wanted to know more about this alternative approach to wellness.

A Gathering of Angels: A Ritual of Preparation for Surgery

Call your friends together before the surgery date. It can be at your home or any place that feels safe and secure. I highly recommend raising some healing energy at the home of the person who is to undergo the surgery, as it will create an aura of restoration. Ask each person to bring something to comfort, reassure, and cure the celebrant: soup, fixings, a soothing eye pillow, sleep balm, a hand-knitted scarf for warmth, body lotion, herbal teas, books, or lavender-infused slippers are all wonderful gifts.

Form a circle of care around the celebrant and light candles. Unscented soy candles are probably best for health reasons. As you go around the circle, ask each person to give his or her gift of caring to the celebrant and say what it represents.

> *I give you this herbal tea mix so you can sip tea and draw from it healing and heat.*

I give you all my love and healing energy and I know you will come back from the hospital healthier than ever before.

The ritual continues until everyone has had a turn to speak and healing gifts and loving energy surround the celebrant. I suggest giving the celebrant hankies beforehand, as I know I myself could not stop my tears of joy. It is completely up to the celebrant to say or do whatever she or he feels during the ritual. In many cases, they may say nothing due to the intensity of this event.

Personal Rituals for Renewal

Every day, you can renew your own health and wellness in many small ways. A cup of green tea with a morning prayer can be a simple ritual that gives you serenity and builds bodily strength. Create and incorporate some personal rituals for your own renewal.

Body Healing Blessing

As I mentioned, I have undergone several surgeries, and, although support and positive "vibes" surrounded me, I was also very scared and had to overcome the possibility of viewing my body as a battleground. In my case, I had to look at my body, and instead of feeling horrified, betrayed, or angry, I had to work hard to feel love for it. I could feel the change in my attitude, and it helped enormously in the long run. I frequently performed self-healing rituals such as the Body Purification Ritual Rub, which is a real boost to body and soul.

Body Purification Ritual Rub

Since the time of the ancients in the Mediterranean and in Mesopotamia, salts from the sea combined with soothing oils have been used to purify the body by way of gentle ritual rubs. From Bathsheba to Cleopatra, these natural salts have been used to smooth the skin and enhance circulation, which is vital to overall body health as the skin is the single largest organ. Salts from the Dead Sea have long been a popular export and are readily available at most health food stores. You can make your own salts, however, and not only control the quality and customize the scent, but save money, too. The definitive benefits that is far and above cost saving is that you can imbue the concoction with your intention, which is absolutely imperative when you are performing rites of self-healing. Cook up your own "kitchen cupboard cure."

Shekinah's Salts

Shekinah translates as "She who dwells within" and is the Hebrew name for the female aspect of God. Legend has it that she co-created the world side by side with Yahweh, the god of Israel. This simple recipe for salts calls up the scents and primal memories of what the Edenic paradise must have been like. A real plus to this recipe is that you can change the essential oils to suit your needs and mood.

The ingredients for the recipe are as follows:

- 3 cups Epsom salts
- ½ cup sweet almond oil
- 1 tablespoon glycerin
- 4 drops ylang-ylang essential oil
- 1 drop jasmine essential oil
- 1 drop clary sage essential oil

Mix well and store in a colored and well-capped glass bottle. You can use these special Shekinah salts in your ritual rub.

Centering: Getting Grounded in Yourself

The best way to prepare for personal ritual is to center yourself. I call this "doing a readjustment," and I believe this is especially important in our overscheduled and busy world. Doing a readjustment helps pull you back into yourself and gets your priorities back on track. Only when you are truly centered can you do the true inner work of self-development that is at the core of ritual.

Centering takes many forms. Experiment on your own to find out what works best for you. My friend Kat Sanborn, for example, does a quick meditation that she calls "the chakra check-in." As previously outlined in this chapter, the chakra system comprises energy points in the astral body associated with various endocrine glands in the physical body. My friend closes her eyes and sits lotus-fashion (ideal if possible, but if you are on a bus or in a meeting you can do this centering exercise just sitting down with your feet on the floor) and visualizes the light and color of each chakra. She visualizes each chakra and mentally runs energy up and down her spine, from bottom to top, pausing at each chakra point. After she does this a few times, a soothing calm surrounds her. I have seen her perform her "chakra check-in" at trade shows and in hotel lobbies, surrounded by the hubbub of many people. She is an ocean of calm at the center of a storm. By working with your chakras, you can become much more in touch with your body and soul.

Prior to performing a ritual, try this centering exercise. Take a comfortable sitting position and find your pulse. Keep your fingers on your pulse point in your wrist until you feel the steady rhythm of your own heart.

Now begin slowly breathing in rhythm with your heartbeat. Inhale for four beats, hold for four beats, and then exhale for five beats. Repeat this pattern for six cycles. People have reported that although it seems hard to match up with the heartbeat at first, with a little bit of practice, your breath and heartbeat will synchronize. Your entire body will relax, and all physical functions will seem slower and more natural than ever before. Another excellent way to center is to light a candle and meditate on it. By focusing on the flame, you bring your being and awareness into focus and come into present time.

Personal Pilgrimage—How to Walk the Labyrinth

The labyrinth represented wholeness to the ancients, combining the circle and the spiral in one archetypal image. The labyrinth is unicursal, meaning there is only one path in and one path out. Put simply, it is a journey into the self, into your own center, and back into the world again. As a prayer and meditation tool, labyrinths are peerless; they awaken intuition.

Do your best to relax before you enter. Deep breaths will help a great deal. If you have a specific question in mind, think it or whisper it to yourself. You will meet others on the pilgrim's path as you are walking; simply step aside and let them continue on their journey as you do the same. The three stages of the labyrinth walk are as follows:

Purification: Here is where you free your mind of all worldly concerns. It is a release, a letting go. Still your mind and open your heart. Shed worries and emotion as you step out on the path.

Illumination: When you have come to the center, you are in the place of illumination. Here, you should stay as long as you feel the need to pray and meditate. In this quiet center, the heart of the labyrinth, you will receive messages from the Divine or from your own higher power. Illumination can also come from deep inside yourself.

Union: This last phase is where you will experience union with the Divine. Lauren Artress says that as you "walk the labyrinth, you become more empowered to find and do the work you feel your soul requires."

Walking Meditation

This is the simplest of rituals you can do every day of your life. As you walk, take the time to look and really *see* what is in your path. For example, my friend Eileen takes a bag with her and picks up every piece of garbage in her path. She does this as an act of love for the earth. During the ten years I have known her, she has probably turned a mountain of litter into recycled glass, paper, and plastic. Goddess bless! This is one type of walking meditation. This very simple daily ritual honors the earth and helps preserve life for all beings.

Color Connection

Color is a form of energy that can be broken down by individual vibrations. We use colors in our homes and at work to affect moods. The right colors can calm, energize, or even romanticize a setting. Colors promote many desired states of being. Anyone using color is tuning in to the vibration frequency of that particular color. Some psychics have the skills and training to read your aura; they can literally see the colors of the energy radiating out from your body.

Other colors not in the spectrum exist in metals, crystals, and stones, and are significant in their own right: brown, gray, black, white, silver, and gold.

❧ **Brown:** the color of humility and poverty; it represents safety and the home and is also often associated with agriculture and grounding.

❧ **Gray:** the color of grief and mourning; it symbolized resurrection in medieval times. Gray is the first color the human eye can perceive in infancy.

❧ **Black:** protection and strength; it fortifies your personal energies and gives them more inner authority. Black symbolizes fertile, life-giving, rich earth, and nourishing rain in Africa.

❧ **White:** purity, peace, patience, and protection; some cultures associate white with death.

❧ **Silver:** relates to communication and greater access to the universe; it indicates a lunar connection or female energy.

❧ **Gold:** direct connection to God or the sun; it facilitates wealth and ease.

The color spectrum is correlated with seven basic vibrations. These are the same vibrations that comprise the musical scale, and the same vibrations that are the foundation of our seven-vibration chakra system. The "lightest" vibrations are at the top and the "heaviest" vibrations are at the bottom. You may recall from earlier in this book that the color system is composed of seven colors, all visible in the rainbow—red, orange, yellow, green, blue, indigo, and violet. A great way to remember the colors is by their collective acronym, which sounds like a name when the letters are strung together: Roy

G. Biv. Consult the following color guide when you are choosing a color for any aspect of your life.

Color management can help you on the most basic level each day. To combat feeling depressed, wear yellow to raise your energy level. If you have a business meeting and you want to put your colleagues at ease, wear earthy colors like brown or green. You can experiment with different combinations, too. Remember, the purpose here is to find your soul colors.

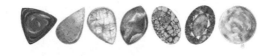

Seven sacred stones

Color Guide

Color: Red
Soul: Passionate and intense
Healing Characteristics and Associations: Security and survival; matters of the body; strong physical connection

Color: Rose Red
Chakra: Root
Soul: Loving
Healing Characteristics and Associations:
Motherhood, home, grounding, money
Crystal Connection: Red gems and crystals aid in matters of the body. Jasper, amber, and agate in shades of red can help shy people feel stronger.

Color: Clear Red
Soul: Angry
Healing Characteristics and Associations: Related to sense of smell

Color: Red Orange
Soul: Passionate
Healing Characteristics and Associations: Sexual Passion

Color: Red Coral
Soul: Vitality
Healing Characteristics and Associations: Skeleton and bones

Color: Pink
Soul: Nurturer
Healing Characteristics and Associations: Boosts self-esteem

Color: Orange
Chakra: Sacral
Soul: Ambitious
Healing Characteristics and Associations: Hunger and sex; lucidity and orderliness; potency and immunity; stimulation and motivation
Crystal Connection: Orange stones can help you focus and build energy.

Color: Yellow
Chakra: Solar Plexus
Soul: Intellectual

Healing Characteristics and Associations: Personal power, freedom, control; fire; the eyes; mental activity
Crystal Connection: Yellow stones such as citrine carry healing energy and can help with nightmares and indigestion.

Color: Green
Chakra: Heart
Soul: Caring nurturer and healer
Healing Characteristics and Associations: Relationships; the heart and lungs; the element of air; sense of touch; will to live; balance of overall health
Crystal Connection: Green stones such as emeralds can represent healing and salvation, as well as closely guarded secrets; green is also the color associated with the Eastern element of wood in Chinese astrology.

Color: Blue
Chakra: Throat
Soul: Teacher
Healing Characteristics and Associations: Communication, listening; intuition; the ears; creativity and mind control
Crystal Connection: Blue stones help maintain calm and protect the aura.

Color: Indigo
Chakra: Third Eye/Intuition
Soul: Spiritual Growth
Healing Characteristics and Associations: Opens third eye; promotes clear-headedness
Crystal Connection: Indigo stones can aid in psychic work.

Color: Violet
Chakra: Crown/Entire Universe
Soul: Deep connection to the spirit
Healing Characteristics and Associations: Helps clear deep pain; works on deep tissue, hypersensitivity; promotes stability and contentment; secrecy
Crystal Connection: Amethysts are good for sensitivity issues. They keep one's energy from draining away. Purplish agates guard stability and contentment.

Ganesha Mudras

Elephant-headed Ganesha is the Indian god who helps overcome all obstacles. What better way to start the New Year that with this mighty deity at your side? Ganesha is beloved in India, where he is also called *Vighnaharta*, the "Lord and Destroyer of Obstacles." When people seek success in work or school, they turn to this jolly elephant god. I keep a little bronze statue of a supine Ganesha on my computer.

Mudra is a type of yoga you do with your hands. It is also called "finger power points." This is a portable yoga that you can do anywhere—on the bus, on the phone, at your desk, even walking down the street. This is a marvelous way to calm yourself and handle stress. Buddha statues are usually shown with the hands in a *mudra* position.

The very easy *Ganesha mudra* begins with you holding your left hand in front of your chest with the palm facing outward, away from your body. Bend your fingers. Grasp your left fingers with your right finders bent, toward your body. Move the hands to the level of your heart, right in front of your chest. Exhale vigorously and gently try to pull your hands apart without releasing the grip. This will create tensions in your upper arms and chest area, exercising those muscles.

Now relax those muscles while inhaling. Repeat these steps six times, then place both your hands on your sternum in the Ganesha clasping position. Note the energy and heat you feel in your body. Now repeat six times with your hands facing in the reversed positions.

The *Ganesha mudra* opens the fourth chakra and gives us "heart"—courage, confidence, and good feelings toward others. It opens us up to fresh encounters and positive new experiences. Performed once a day, this is a marvelous way to strengthen your upper body. It is also believed to open the bronchial tubes and stimulate the lung area.

Use the rituals in this chapter to become one with yourself and find peace within. May you use this learned tranquility to better participate in other rituals that focus on important aspects of your life.

Ayurveda is the ancient Indian "Science of Life" that has become very popular in the past few years, Aromatic plants and the oils derived from them are a major part of this wellness wisdom tradition. Herbaceous species used for ayurvedic healing include tulsi (holy basil), coriander, fennel, and various sages and mints, as well as aromatic roots including vetiver, valerian, and calamus. Ayurvedic flowers include roses, jasmine, champa, marigolds, and lotuses. Woody and tree species include agar, cedar, eucalyptus, pine, and sandalwood. Fragrant resins are utilized, including frankincense and myrrh. As you might expect, Ayurveda is also rich in spices, including cinnamon, cardamom, black pepper, long pepper, ginger, nutmeg, and clove. Several aromatic grasses, such as lemongrass, are found in the tradition as well.

Your Chakras

First Chakra—Patchouli Grounds Your Root Chakra

Patchouli balances the root chakra at the base of your spine. Represented by the color red and associated with the then physical element of earth, the root chakra is about grounding to the physical world and basic survival and self-preservation. Using patchouli will enable you to be grounded and have more stability, stillness, prosperity, and robust health, as well as a sense of safety and security. This essential oil also helps you overcome fatigue and feeling down.

Second Chakra—Neroli Balances Your Sacral Chakra

Neroli essential oil stabilizes the sacral chakra, which is located in the lower abdomen between the pelvis and the navel center, a few inches below the belly button. Associated with the element of water and the color orange, it represents vitality and passion and is associated with the sacral vertebra as well as the reproductive organs and the body's circulatory system. A balanced sacral chakra carries the following characteristics: ability to enjoy pleasure, emotional intelligence, sexual satisfaction, passion, and the ability to embrace change. This essential oil brings the energy of pure love and lightness of being, driving away sorrows and bringing a peaceful, stable sense of calm. Neroli also opens you to love within yourself and the freedom of allowing love to flow freely.

Third Chakra—Pine Invigorates Your Solar Plexus Chakra

Pine essential oil is connected to the solar plexus chakra, which is located above the navel and correlates with the color yellow and the element of fire. The solar plexus chakra represents willpower, motivation, and vigor and is associated with the pancreas, liver, spleen, stomach, lower back muscles, and the metabolism and digestion. A balanced solar plexus chakra gives rise to confidence, warmth, self-discipline, steadiness, and a positive sense of self. Pine essential oil is an oil for the restoration of the heart when your emotions have become hard or jaded. This oil releases you from old wounds, letting you move forward without the baggage of the past and bringing the ability to experience your emotions in real time versus playing out echoes from the past. This oil allows you to move forward. You will feel replenished and new, which will allow you to bring growth and inner peace to your future relationships.

Fourth Chakra—Rose Oil Opens Your Heart Chakra

Rose essential oil will open and balance your heart chakra and bring self-acceptance and love into your life. This chakra center is associated with the color green and the element of air, and it is related to the lymph glands, heart, rib cage, lungs, skin, arms, hands, circulation, and the immune system. A balanced heart chakra will lead to the following characteristics in an individual: healthy self-esteem, contentment, compassion, acceptance, and peace of mind. Use rose essential oil's scent for releasing blocked feelings stored in the chest, internalized grief, melancholy, and repressed emotions.

Fifth Chakra—Lavender Aids Your Throat Chakra

Lavender essential oil is connected to the throat chakra, which correlates to the colors blue or turquoise and the element of spirit or ether. The throat chakra is about speaking, self-expression, and communication and is associated with the thyroid, esophagus, neck, shoulders, arms, hands, and the sense of hearing. A balanced throat chakra will support the following characteristics: clear communication with others and self, good listening skills, good sense of time, and a full voice. Lavender essential oil brings spiritual growth by helping you integrate your experiences, bringing an expanded awareness and perspective. This oil will help you communicate more effectively.

Sixth Chakra—Sandalwood Awakens Your Third Eye Chakra

The third eye chakra is located in the middle of the forehead and is represented by the color indigo and the element of light. The third eye chakra represents self-reflection and knowledge. It is also associated with the pituitary gland, left brain hemisphere, left eye, nose, ears, sinuses, conscious mind, the endocrine system, neurological system, and small muscle control. A balanced third eye chakra will yield strong intuition, good memory, ease remembering dreams, the ability to visualize, and a guiding vision for life. Sandalwood essential oil abets meditation and is used by healers and spiritual leaders worldwide as it brings an inner awareness and sense of ease in engaging with higher consciousness. Sandalwood helps break down illusions, helping you align with your most authentic self.

Seventh Chakra—Lime Energizes Your Crown Chakra

Lime essential oil is for the crown chakra at the very top of your head. Represented by violet and the element of thought, this chakra is the center of self-knowledge, self-will, and divine connection. It is associated with the pineal gland, pituitary gland, cerebral cortex, cerebrum, the right eye, the right brain hemisphere, the central nervous system, the subconscious mind, and large muscle control. A balanced crown chakra will produce wisdom, intelligence, the ability to analyze, spiritual connection, and open mindedness. Lime is a great essential oil to use for cutting and detaching energy cords that no longer serve you. This oil is useful for enhancing your perception of the truth inside any situation. It allows you to release any illusion that you may have confused with reality.

Here are a few more suggestions:

- Root Chakra: Cypress
- Sacral Chakra: Ylang-ylang
- Solar Plexus Chakra: Ginger
- Heart Chakra: Jasmine
- Throat Chakra: Roman Chamomile
- Third Eye Chakra: Rosemary
- Crown Chakra: Frankincense

CHAPTER NINE

Herbal Detox for Your Home for a Happy Healthy Family

Your home should feel good from the minute you walk in and every moment you spend in your own domain. Positive energy at home goes hand-in-hand with purification. One of the greatest tools for purification is sage. While every metaphysical store has it in quantity, I highly recommend gathering or growing sage yourself. Aromatic sage dries quickly and can be bound into thick "smudge sticks," which you should keep at the ready in a fireproof clay dish. To make a smudge stick, take dried sage leaves and bind them with green and gold thread wound nine times around the bundle and knotted at each loop. Leave room for a handle at the base of the wand, where you wind and knot the green and gold threads thrice more. This will honor the three Fates who hold the thread of our destiny in their hands: Clotho spins the thread of life; Lachesis chooses its length and outcome; and Atropos cuts the thread.

Use your smudge stick at any time purification is in order, especially if you've moved, started a new job, bought a new car, or purchased any second-hand clothing or furniture. This will help remove any energy that might be clinging from the previous owner; it can also be useful to smudge items bought new to clear random energies from them. If have just performed a big decluttering in your home or office, you can further cleanse your personal space by smudging it with sage smoke.

Light your smudge stick; moving clockwise, circle the area or items to be purified, gently moving the smudge stick so that the purifying smoke is wafted into various corners.

Give a lot of thought to what constructive changes you wish to see in your life or what positive qualities you want to develop further in yourself.

For example, right now, I want to get even more organized, so I will get some lazulite. Crystals and sacred stones can be a great source of clarity and help with processing emotions. Of course, getting organized requires some letting go and getting rid of belongings that have seen better days. This used to be a real problem for me. As any of my friends can tell you, my cozy cottage is lined with magazines, journals, and books, books, books! But I *really* feel the need to declutter my life and streamline it—get a bit more Zen. So, I'll have to get organized with lazulite power and then let go with lepidolite! Also, I have never really had any jade, but recently, I feel like I need the grounding and stabilizing effects of this stone. Additionally, I need to get more prosperity-minded. I need to be better about saving money and thinking in terms of my future security so I'm not reading tarot out on the sidewalk when I'm ninety! In light of this, I have been walking through San Francisco's Chinatown and feeling very attracted to different jades. I'm sure you feel such urges and attractions, too. Often, this might be your subconscious giving you a gentle nudge about some growing you need to do. Listen to those inner voices, and you will reap the benefits again and again.

Change Your Life with Sacred Stones

- ≫ **amber** for grounding
- ≫ **aventurine** for creative visualization
- ≫ **bloodstone** for abundance and prosperity
- ≫ **carnelian** for opening doors for you your family
- ≫ **citrine** for getting motivated and attracting money and success
- ≫ **geode** for getting through periods of extreme difficulty
- ≫ **hematite** for strength and courage
- ≫ **jasper** for stability
- ≫ **rhodochrosite** for staying on course with your life's true purpose
- ≫ **watermelon tourmaline** for help with planning your best possible future

Ritual for Letting Go

Truth be told, many of us have hoarded to some extent in our lives. I joke to my friends and family that I have "paper issues" with all my books and magazines, but I also amass colored glass vases and bottles, interesting chairs, and quirky candleholders. And much more. At a certain point, I realized that things had gotten out of control and that what had once been an interesting collection of "objets" was quickly headed toward "Cat Lady Hoarder Next Door." When I really looked at my home, I knew I needed to give away a lot of things I didn't really even *see* anymore. Nevertheless, it's hard. We love our shiny objects! The following spell for letting go will transform both you and your home.

Rite for Releasing

Take a few of the items you are giving away (selling on eBay is a good idea, too!) and place them on a little table, then put the table somewhere near the front door. You are setting up a temporary altar. Gather a white candle, copal incense, and a sage leaf in a white dish, along with a small white sheet of paper and a black pen.

Light the candle and the incense and intone:

> *As I walk in wisdom, this I know,*
> *Material goods are meant to flow.*
> *I rid myself of blocks so I can grow.*
> *With this rite, I am letting go!*
> *And so it is.*

Take each item and name it as you release it; for example, "Purple dish, with grace and gratitude, I let you go!" Make a brief note of each possession to be released on the piece of paper.

After you have recorded all the items, read your list aloud, then carefully light the piece of paper and burn it in the white dish while repeating the spell words above. When the paper has burned to ash, snuff the candle while the ashes cool down completely. Take the dish outside the door and toss the thoroughly cooled ashes into the air and wind. Now, go back in and pack up the newly released items and get them out of your house into the trunk of your car, a storage shed, or the nearest Goodwill or recycling/reuse center. The important thing is to get all those things out of your house so the energy flow inside is improved. If you moved bigger pieces such as shelves or chairs, I highly recommend a ritual floor wash. Once you have done that, the energy in your home will shimmer and sparkle with freshness!

Peppermint Clove Ghostbuster Spray

To rid a house of haunting intrusions, brew a peppermint and clove tea infusion. Lightly spray the potion throughout the space, and out, out, the ghost will race. Burning frankincense and myrrh incense sends negative spirits flying away as well.

Eco-Detergents and Nontoxic Paint

We all want to live in an enchanted cottage, a charming residence in every sense of the word. Several years ago, I learned that all the chemicals in our conventional cleansing products introduce potential toxins into our lives, along with a certain amount of negative energy. Who likes the smell of raw bleach, over-perfumed detergents, and those scary oven cleaners? They strip away the natural and are simply too harsh. It is even a danger to have them around young children whose curiosity could lead them into trouble. I think we can all agree it makes a lot of sense to simply not have anything in your kitchen cabinet that is marked "poisonous." There are so many options that are inexpensive and will make your home and anyone who walks in the door feel healthier and happier. Creating your own all-organic green witchery cleaners gives you the opportunity to put the *most magic* into every surface, room, and corner of your home. Every time your home is cleaned using these pagan potions, you are bettering the vibrations of your home, creating healing energy, eliminating toxins and introducing a light, bright positivity right where you live. There is no more powerful enchantment than this; it is the foundation for a peaceful and pleasurable home.

DIY All-Purpose Cottage Cleaner

- 1 Teaspoon baking soda
- 1 Teaspoon liquid Castile soap

- ≫ 3 drops lemon essential oil or 1 teaspoon lemon juice

- ≫ 1 quart warm water

Pour the above into a bowl and mix well; transfer to a clean spray bottle and shake. If you have a tougher job than usual, add a cup of white vinegar to the other ingredients. Baking soda is a mild alkaline abrasive, so don't use it on fine furniture or delicate fabrics. Otherwise, it is quite miraculous for tough stains, rust, ovens, tiles, stain removal, tough greases, smelly fridges, and so many other household chores.

Love Your Linens and They'll Love You Back: Secrets of Stain Removal

If you spill coffee or red wine on your couch, carpet, or tablecloth, pour plain table salt into the spill and it will soak the staining liquid right up. The salt turning purplish blue as it soaks up red wine is truly spellbinding! Vacuum it up and the stain will be gone.

Stained clothes, linens, and such should be soaked in cold water with either baking soda or white vinegar, and then washed in cold water only to avoid setting the stain.

There is no need to use bleach in your laundry; for white fabric, use a cup of Borax in your load.

Good for Wood Eco Floor Cleaner

Combine the following in a big bowl:

- ≫ 1 tablespoon white vinegar

- 1 tablespoon olive oil
- 5 drops lemon essential oil
- 1 quart warm water

Mix everything together, preferably in a glass bowl, and pour into a clean spray bottle. As always, use caution even with these homely, organic ingredients and avoid getting vinegar, lemon juice, Borax, or any of your eco witchery concoctions in your eyes. Simply aim the spray at your floor and mop with a clean damp mop. Follow by mopping with hot water. Allow the floor to dry a bit and buff with clean dry cloths into which you have sprinkled a few drops of lavender oil. Your floors will look really good and smell even better.

Floral Floor Cleansing

I haven't used store-bought cleansers since the year 2004, when a health challenge awakened me to the importance of ridding my environment of any toxins or potentially harmful chemicals. I think it is a very good idea for all of us to consider as our health is precious. I know this made a difference for me and my loved ones. And the smell of a home freshly cleaned with lemons and scentful natural oils feels wonderful.

Gather the following:

- 1 quart of white vinegar
- ⅓ cup of lemon juice
- 8 drops lavender oil
- 3 cinnamon sticks

- ∾ 3 sage leaves

- ∾ 3 mint stems with leaves

- ∾ 1 cup hot water

- ∾ a new mop

In a medium glass mixing bowl, pour the cup of boiling hot water, then add the mint, eight drops of lavender oil, sage leaves, and cinnamon sticks. Stir once and let steep covered for a half hour. After it has finished steeping, stir in the one-third cup of lemon juice.

Take a clean bucket and fill with two gallons of warm water and a quart of white vinegar. Using a kitchen sieve, strain the herbal mix into the bucket and give it a stir with a wooden spoon. If your floor is a delicate or antique and rare wood, leave out the lemon, but otherwise, this is a suitable albeit magical floor wash for any purpose. Take your brand-new mop and dip it into the bucket, wring it out, and clean the floor very thoroughly.

Do-It-Yourself Herbal Homekeeping

Soda Scrub

To make your own all-natural cleaning scrub, try this simple scrubbing paste recipe: mix a half cup of baking soda with liquid castile soap until it's the consistency of frosting. Scrub whatever surface needs cleaning, then rinse with water. Do bear in mind that baking soda is

slightly abrasive so fragile fabrics and surfaces may
not fare well, including glass, mirrors, or antique and
rare woods. You can do a little test on an area that is not
noticeable, and if no issues arise, then scrub a dub to
your heart's content.

No Chemicals Laundry Detergent

Want to get away from the chemicals, foaming agents,
and synthetic fragrances found in most laundry
detergents? Using a box grater to grate a bar of pure
natural soap into a powder. Freeze the soap for super-
fast grating, and then mix the grated powder with one
cup of Borax, one cup of washing soda, and a few drops
of lemon juice (optional) for cold and warm water loads.
Use one to two tablespoons per load.

Tea Tree Clean

Instead of toxic, chemical-laden wipes you get at the
store, make your own to have handy for spills as well as
for scheduled cleanings. Mix one cup of white vinegar,
half a cup of lemon juice, and eight drops of tea tree oil.
Soak clean washcloths or paper towels in the mixture
and store them in a sealable bag; they can last a month
for on-the-go spills.

Natural Cleaning with Vinegar

If I could only use one item to clean my home with, it
would be vinegar. A natural disinfectant that only costs
pennies, vinegar deals with dirt, smells, stains, grease,
and mold—especially in the shower. I've cleaned my

whole house with just a spray bottle of vinegar and a little liquid soap. To make it smell really clean and good, add a few drops of calming lavender oil (also a natural disinfectant), easily found at a reasonable cost at your local health food stores. Just remember, you're not making gallons, you're making a small bottle. Because they contain no preservatives, DIY cleaning mixes don't last very long, so use regularly for a clean green home and then fill your spray bottle anew!

Baking Soda Fresh

Baking soda is wonderful deodorizer around the house and can be used to freshen and launder clothing as well as to freshen furniture or carpets. It can also be used as an eco-friendly oven cleaner. Since the oven is where you cook your food, it's better to skip oven cleaner chemicals, which leave a residue that could be quite unhealthy. Make a paste by adding water, or equal parts water and vinegar, to one cup of baking soda. Coat the inside of the oven and leave overnight. In the morning, turn the oven on low heat for an hour, then let cool. Use a spray bottle of water and vinegar to soften the hardened paste, then use elbow grease to scrub it off. When you are baking that batch of cookies for your loved ones, you can rest assured no fumes are getting into the yummy treats!

Salt Is Magic!

Some people swear by scouring pots, pans, and cooking surfaces with salt. It absorbs oil and grease, making it great for the stovetop, which can have cooking splatters that can be tough to remove. Sprinkle it on and scrub away with a sponge or enamel-safe scrubber.

Lemon Works for Everything

Instead of discarding lemon halves after you've used their juice for cooking or lemonade, save them to use as scrubbers for cleaning wood cutting boards without damaging them. You can also use fresh lemon juice mixed with baking soda to brighten white tiles, sinks, or tubs, or make natural wood polish for floors by mixing a little fresh lemon juice with olive oil. This citrus fruit is a natural lightening agent that you can use in place of bleach, which should be used sparingly, if at all. Throw discolored white socks, towels, or shirts in a stockpot with water and a few used lemons; simmer for a little while to lighten. If you hang them outside to dry, the combination of sunlight and your low-cost lemon whitener will refresh your laundry until it is practically gleaming!

Make cleaning a cheese grater a snap: Take a lemon cut in half and rub it on all the surfaces of a cheese grater. The lemon's acid breaks down the fatty cheese residue on the grater. If cheese is really stuck, here's an extra technique to try: set up a small plate with a layer of table salt on it, then dip the lemon in the salt. Like commercial scrubbing powder (but without all the chemicals), the salt will increase the friction on your grater; together with the lemon, it will effectively remove most stuck-on food.

Takes tarnish off your metal jewelry: Use two tablespoons of lemon juice concentrate to three cups water, then rub jewelry well with a soft cloth. The acidity of the concentrated lemon juice will work to remove tarnish.

Add lemon to food to reduce bacteria: Since bacteria require an alkaline environment to stay alive, add lemon juice or fruit to produce, meat, or even water to slow down microbial growth.

Sanitize your cutting board: Want to deep clean your cutting board without running it through a dishwasher? Putting a wooden cutting board in the dishwasher is just not a good idea, but especially after preparing meat, a natural antibacterial treatment is in order. Rub a cut lemon on your cutting board and let it sit with the lemon juice on it overnight, then rinse it well in the morning. Bacteria will be banished, and your cutting board will have a lemon-fresh aroma.

Restore wooden furniture's natural shine: Combine equal parts of olive oil and lemon juice with a little mayonnaise and stir well. This mixture will both remove previous polish buildup on wood furniture due to the acidity of the citrus and will also condition the wood.

Keep rice from sticking together: Set up your rice pot; while the water is heating, put a teaspoon of lemon juice into the pot and your cooked rice will come out in nice separate grains. Other types of citrus fruit can also be used depending on what type of dish will be served with your grain. Believe it or not, citrus juice also enhances the whiteness of the rice itself.

Degrease pots & pans and stovetop or grill: Cut a lemon in half and dip it in salt as described above for cleaning a cheese grater. When you scrub a copper-bottomed pot with it, tarnish will be removed so quickly you'll swear it's magic. It works wonderfully well to clean the stovetop and barbecue grill, too, as well as stainless steel pots and pans.

Natural weed killer: Don't give in to the marketing of chemical herbicides; besides exposing you and your family to dangerous toxins, they are bad for the planet as well. Combine one part white vinegar with four parts lemon juice in a spray bottle, then give it a good shake and spray your plantings, whether in indoor pots or your garden.

Herbal Wreaths Make a Home

Oftentimes, your kitchen is the heart of the home. Something about cooking and sharing food brings people together. An herbal wreath hanging on the kitchen door can be a source of love and luck. You'll need the following for your creation:

- ⋙ Freshly cut herbs of your choice
- ⋙ A wire wreath frame, available from most craft stores
- ⋙ Either string or florist's wire, ribbon, and a hot glue gun

This is truly one of the simplest craft projects you can ever make; simply use the wreath frame as a base, and use string or the florist's wire to anchor the fresh herbs into place. Finish it off with a colorful ribbon or other magical decorative touches you may want to add.

Curative Wreath: These are the ideal herbs for a wreath that brings curative healing properties: lavender, barley, comfrey, rosemary, peppermint, borage, olive, eucalyptus, and apple blossom. Brown and green ribbon add a touch of healing color.

Security Wreath: Hang a guardian wreath on your front door made with heather, holly, dill, foxglove, garlic, sandalwood, snapdragon, mustard, foxglove, mistletoe, and mugwort. White and blue ribbons add security and serenity.

Prosperity Wreath: Greet prosperity at the door with herbs associated with money magic including clover, chamomile, sunflower, apple, cinnamon, myrtle, basil, and bay leaf. Weave in gold and green ribbons to add to your luck.

Heart Wreath: Don't wait until Valentine's Day to try this; love should be twenty-four-seven, 365. Invite love into your home than by hanging a wreath full of love herbs on your door. Any combination of these will work beautifully, and I recommend using herbs that personally resonate for you among these options: allspice, clove, catnip, fig, bleeding heart, periwinkle, tulip, peppermint, violet, daffodil, lavender, and marjoram to light up your love light. Adorn with pink and red ribbons to let the universe know you're ready to welcome love into your life.

CONCLUSION

The Magic of Herbs and Plants

. . . .

I do love that simple wisdom from the family farm of my childhood can still help people in the high-tech world we live in. I have discovered that the homemade healing potions, teas, and cures our grandmothers cooked up from the kitchen cabinet are the best things to turn to in tough times. There is a veritable cornucopia of cures and pagan prescriptions for you to try herein. I have also dealt with anxiety and issues around grief and loss myself in the past couple of years, so I can offer my own testimonial to the supportive effects of these recipes, rituals, and spells. It is my sincere hope that the suggestions here offer you and your loved ones much relief from any stress and strain you might be experiencing. Keeping your life in balance with nature is of the utmost importance. Taking a walk in the nearest park or even around the block during the workday can be a mindfulness meditation. Mother Nature is the ultimate healer, and spending time outdoors in her abundant beauty will bring you much peace of mind. Practicing the art of sacred self-care will enable you to thrive and stay inspired so you can bring your special magic into the world.

Any good herbal healer knows that the best ingredients can be found in your kitchen or your own backyard. For the more unusual ingredients, try your local health food market, herbalist, or apothecary; also, as interest in things herbal has become more and more mainstream, new online mail-order outlets have, dare I say, mushroomed up. Please be in touch and let us know how the recipes and suggestions herein are working for you. If you like, please share your stories of healing as it would be wonderful to know. Just email info@mango.bz and let us know your thoughts.

Be well; I wish you great good health, much love, and deep happiness!

THE VICTORIAN ART OF FLORIOGRAPHY:

The Meaning of Flowers

. . . .

Several flower dictionaries were written and published in the Victorian era in an effort to preserve the lore handed down through the ages on the meaning of flowers and the properties associated with them. This is known as "floriography," and many a hedgewitch contributed to this body of wisdom for flower magic and herbal healing. Should you wish to favor a friend, family member, or even a new flame with a bouquet, this floral index will guide your choices.

A

Abatina: Fickleness

Acacia: Chaste love

Acacia, Pink: Elegance

Acacia, Yellow: Secret love

Acanthus: The fine arts, artifice

Achillea Millefolia: War

Aconite, Crowfoot: Lustre

Aconite, Wolfsbane: Misanthropy

Adonis: Sorrowful remembrance

African Marigold: Vulgar minds

Agnus Castus: Coldness

Agrimony: Thankfulness, gratitude

Almond: Stupidity, indiscretion

Almond, Flowering: Hope

Almond, Laurel: Perfidy

Allspice: Compassion

Aloe: Grief, affection

Althea Frutex: Persuasion

Alyssum, Sweet: Worth beyond beauty

Amaranth: Immortality, unfading love

Amaranth, Cockscomb: Foppery, affectation

Amaranth, Globe: Unchangeable

Amaryllis: Pride

Ambrosia: Love returned

American Elm: Patriotism

American Linden: Matrimony

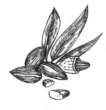

Almonds

B

Bachelor's Buttons: Single blessedness

Balm: Sympathy

Balm, Gentle: Pleasantry

Balm of Gilead: Cure, relief

Balsam: Impatience

Balsam, Red: Touch me not, impatient resolve

Barberry: Sourness, sharpness, ill temper

Basil: Hatred

Bay Leaf: I change but in death

Bay Tree: Glory

Bay Wreath: Reward of merit

Bearded Crepis: Protection

Beech Tree: Prosperity

Bee Orchis: Industry

Bee Ophrys: Error

Begonia: Dark thoughts

Belladonna: Silence

Bell Flower, White: I declare against you

Betony: Surprise

Bilberry: Treachery

Bindweed, Great: Insinuation

Bindweed, Small: Humility

Birch: Meekness

Birdsfoot Trefoil: Revenge

Bitterweed, Nightshade: Truth

Black Poplar: Courage

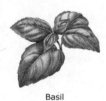

Basil

C

Cabbage: Profit

Cacalia: Adulation

Calceolaria: Keep this for my sake

Calla Aethiopica: Magnificent beauty

Calycanthus: Benevolence

Camellia Japonica, White: Unpretending excellence

Chamomile: Energy in adversity

Campanula: Gratitude

Canariensis: Self-esteem

Canary Grass: Perseverance

Candytuft: Indifference

Canterbury Bell: Acknowledgement

Cardamine: Paternal error

Cardinal Flower: Distinction

Carnation, Red: Alas for my poor heart

Carnation, Striped: Refusal

Carnation, Yellow: Disdain

Catsus: Warmth

Catchfly: Snare

Catchfly, Red: Youthful love

Catchfly, White: Betrayal

Cedar: Strength

Cedar of Lebanon: Incorruptible

Cedar Leaf: I live for thee

Celandine: Joys to come

Centuary: Felicity

Cerebus, Creeping: Modest genius

Champignon: Suspicion

Crown, Imperial: Majesty, powerful

D, E

Daffodil: Regard

Daffodil, Great Yellow: Chivalry

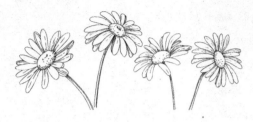

Daisies

Dahlia, Single: Good taste

Dahlia: Instability

Daisy, Double: Participation

Daisy, Garden: I share your sentiment

Daisy, One-Eyed: A token

Daisy, Particolored: Beauty

Daisy, Red: Unconscious

Daisy, White: Innocent

Daisy, Wild: I will think of it

Dandelion: Oracle

Daphne Odora: Painting the lily

Darnel: Vice

Dead Leaves: Sadness

Dew Plant: A serenade

Diosma: Uselessness

Dittany of Crete: Birth

Dittany, White: Passion

Dock: Patience

Dodder of Thyme: Baseness

Dogsbane: Deceit, falsehood

Dogwood: Durability

Dragon Plant: Snare

Dragonwort: Horror

Dried Flax: Utility

Ebony Tree: Blackness

Eglantine or Sweet Briar: Poetry, I wound to heal

Elder: Zealousness

Elm: Dignity

Enchanter's Nightshade: Fascination, witchcraft

Endive: Frugality

Eschscholtzia: Sweetness

Eupatorium: Delay

Evergreen: Poverty

Evergreen, Thorn: Solace in adversity

Everlasting Pea: Lasting pleasure, an appointed meeting

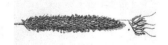

Foxtail

F, G

Fennel: Worthy of all praise

Fern, Flowering: Fascination

Fern: Sincerity

Ficoides, Ice Plant: Your looks freeze me

Fig: Argument

Fig, Marigold: Idleness

Fig Tree: Prolific

Flax: Fate, domestic industry, I feel your kindness

Flax-leaved Golden Locks: Tardiness

Fleur-de-lis: Flame

Fleur-de-Luce: Confidence in heaven

Flower-of-an-Hour: Delicate beauty

Fly Orchis: Error

Fly Trap: Deceit

Fools Parsley: Silliness

Forget-Me-Not: True love

Foxglove: Insincerity

Foxtail Grass: Sporting

French Honeysuckle: Rustic beauty

French Marigold: Jealousy

Frog Ophrys: Disgust

Fritillary, Checquered: Persecution

Fullers Teasel: Misanthropy, importunity

Fumitory: Spleen

Fuschia, Scarlet: Taste

Furze or Gorse: Enduring affection

Garden Anemone: Forsaken

Garden Chervil: Sincerity

Garden Marigold: Uneasiness

Garden Ranunculus: You are rich in attractions

Garden Sage: Esteem

Garland of Roses: Reward of virtue

Gentian: You are unjust

Germander Speedwell: Facility

Geranium, Dark: Melancholy

Geranium, Ivy: Bridal favor

Geranium, Nutmeg: An expected meeting

Geranium, Oak-leaved: True friendship

Geranium, Pencil-leaved: Ingenuity

Geranium, Rose or Pink: Preference

Geranium, Scarlet: Comforting

Geranium, Silver-leaved: Recall

Geranium, Wild: Steadfast piety

Gillyflower: Lasting beauty

Gladiolus: Strength of character

Glory Flower: Glorious beauty

Gloxinia: A proud spirit

Goats Rue: Reason

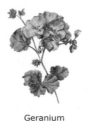

Geranium

H, I, J

Hand Flower Tree: Warming

Harebell: Submission, grief

Hawkweed: Quick-sightedness

Hawthorne: Hope

Hazel: Reconciliation

Heartsease or Pansy: You occupy my thoughts

Heath: Solitude

Helenium: Tears

Heliotrope: Devotion

Hellebore: Scandal, calumny

Hemlock: You will be my death

Hemp: Fate

Henbane: Imperfection

Hepatica: Confidence

Hibiscus: Delicate beauty

Holly: Foresight

Holly Herb: Enchantment

Hollyhock: Fecundity

Honesty: Honesty, sincerity

Honey Flower: Love sweet and secret

Honeysuckle: Bonds of love, sweetness of disposition

Honeysuckle, Coral: The color of my fate

Honeysuckle, French: Rustic beauty

Hop: Injustice

Hornbeam: Ornament

Hortensia: You are cold

Houseleek: Vivacity, domestic economy

Houstonia: Content

Hoya: Sculpture

Humble Plant: Despotism

Hyacinth: Sport, game, play

Hyacinth, Blue: Constancy

Hyacinth, Purple: Sorrow

Hyacinth, White: Unobtrusiveness, loveliness

Hydrangea: A boaster, heartlessness

Hyssop: Cleanliness

Iceland Moss: Health

Ice Plant: Your looks freeze me

Imperial Montaque: Power

Indian Cress: Warlike trophy

Indian Pink, Double: Always lovely

Indian Plum: Privation

Iris: Message

Iris, German: Flame

Ivy: Friendship, fidelity

Ivy, Sprig of with tendrils: Assiduous to please

Jacobs Ladder: Come down

Japan Rose: Beauty is your only attraction

Jasmine, Cape: Transport of joy

Jasmine, Carolina: Separation

Jasmine, Indian: Attachment

Jasmine, Spanish: Sensuality

Jasmine, Yellow: Grace and elegance

Jasmine, White: Amiability

Jonquil: I desire a return of affection

Judas Tree: Unbelief, betrayal

Justicia: The perfection of female loveliness

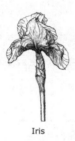

Iris

K, L

Kennedya: Mental beauty

King-Cups: Desire of riches

Laburnum: Forsaken, pensive beauty

Lady's Slipper: Capricious beauty

Lagerstromia, Indian: Eloquence

Lantana: Rigor

Larch: Audacity, boldness

Larkspur: Lightness, levity

Larkspur, Pink: Fickleness

Larkspur, Purple: Haughtiness

Laurel: Glory

Laurel, Common, in flower: Perfidy

Laurel, Ground: Perseverance

Laurel, Mountain: Ambition

Laurestina: A token

Lavender: Distrust

Leaves, Dead: Melancholy

Lemon: Zest

Lemon Blossoms: Fidelity in love

Lent Lilly: Sweet disposition

Lettuce: Cold-heartedness

Lichen: Dejection, solitude

Lilac, Field: Humility

Lilac, Purple: First emotions of love

Lilac, White: Youthful innocence

Lily, Day: Coquetry

Lily, Yellow: Falsehood, gaiety

Lily of the Valley: Return of happiness

Linden or Lime Tree: Conjugal love

Lint: I feel my obligation

Liquorice, Wild: I declare against you

Live Oak: Liberty

Liverwort: Confidence

Lobelia: Malevolence

Locust Tree: Elegance

Locust Tree, Green: Affection beyond the grave

London Pride: Frivolity

Lote Tree: Concord

Lotus: Eloquence

Lotus Flower: Estranged love

Lotus Leaf: Recantation

Love-in-a-Mist: Perplexity

Love-Lies-Bleeding: Hopeless, not heartless

Lucerne: Life

Lupin: Voraciousness

Lotus flower

M, N, O

Madder: Calumny

Magnolia: Love of nature

Magnolia, Laurel-leaved: Dignity

Magnolia, Swamp: Perseverance

Mallow: Mildness

Mallow, Marsh: Beneficence

Mallow, Syrian: Consumed by love

Mallow, Venetian: Delicate beauty

Manchineel Tree: Falsehood

Mandrake: Horror

Maple: Reserve

Marigold: Grief, despair

Marigold, African: Vulgar minds

Marigold, French: Jealousy

Marigold, Prophetic: Prediction

Marjoram: Blushes

Marvel of Peru: Timidity

Meadow Lychnis: Wit

Meadow Saffron: My best days are past

Meadowsweet: Uselessness

Mercury: Goodness

Mesembryanthemum: Idleness

Mezereon: Desire to please

Michaelmas Daisy: Afterthought

Mignonette: Your qualities surpass your charms

Milfoil: War

Milkvetch: Your presence softens my pains

Milkwort: Hermitage

Mimosa, Sensitive Plant: Sensitiveness

Mint: Virtue

Mistletoe: I surmount difficulties

Narcissus: Egotism

Narcissus, Double: Female ambition

Nasturtium: Patriotism

Nemophila: I forgive you

Nettle, Common Stinging: You are cruel

Nettle, Burning: Slander

Night-blooming Cereus: Transient beauty

Night Convolvulus: Night

Nightshade: Falsehood

Oak Leaves: Bravery

Oak Tree: Hospitality

Oats: The witching soul of music

Oleander: Beware

Olive: Peace

Orange Blossoms: Bridal festivities, your purity equals your loveliness

Orange Flowers: Chastity

Orange Tree: Generosity

Orchid: A belle

Osier: Frankness

Osmunda: Dreams

Ox Eye: Patience

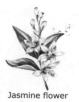

Jasmine flower

P, Q, R

Palm: Victory

Pansy: Thoughts

Parsley: Festivity

Pasque Flower: You have no claims

Patience Dock: Patience

Passion Flower: Religious superstition

Pea, Everlasting: An appointed meeting, lasting pleasure

Pea, Sweet: Departure, lasting pleasures

Peach: Your qualities like your charms are unequalled

Peach Blossom: I am your captive

Quaking Grass: Agitation

Quamoclit: Busybody

Queen's Rocket: You are the Queen of Coquettes; passion

Quince: Temptation

Ragged Robin: Wit

Ranunculus: You are radiant with charms

Ranunculus, Garden: You are rich in all relations

Ranunculus, Wild: Ingratitude

Raspberry: Remorse

Rye Grass, Darnel: Vice

Red Catchfly: Youthful love

Reed: Complaisance, music

Reed, Split: Indiscretion

Rhododendron, Rosebay: Danger, beware

Rhubarb: Advice

Rocket: Rivalry

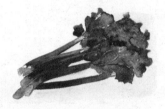

Rhubarb

S

Saffron: Beware of success

Saffron, Crocus: Mirth

Saffron, Meadow: My happiest days are past

Sage: Domestic virtue

Sage, Garden: Esteem

Sainfoin: Agitation

Saint John's Wort: Animosity

Salvia, Blue: I think of you

Salvia, Red: Forever thine

Saxifrage, Mossy: Affection

Scabicus: Unfortunate love

Scarlet Lychnis: Sunbeaming eyes

Schinus: Religious enthusiasm

Scilla, Blue: Forgive and forget

Scilla, Sibirica: Pleasure without alloy

Scilla, White: Sweet innocence

Scotch Fir: Elevation

Sensitive Plant: Sensibility

Shamrock: Light-heartedness

Snakesfoot: Horror

Snowball: Bound

Snowdragon: Presumption

Snowdrop: Hope

Sorrel: Affection

Sorrel, Wild: Wit, ill-timed

Sorrel, Wood: Joy

Stephanotis: You can boast too much

Stock, Ten Week: Promptness

Stonecrop: Tranquility

Straw, Broken: Rupture of a contract

Straw, Whole: Union

Strawberry Blossom: Foresight

Strawberry Tree: Esteem, not love

Sumac, Venice: Splendor

Sunflower, Dwarf: Adoration

Sunflower, Tall: Haughtiness

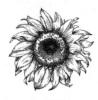

Sunflower

T

Tamarisk: Crime

Tansy, Wild: I declare war against you

Teasel: Misanthropy

Tendrils of Climbing Plants: Ties

Thistle, Common: Austerity

Thistle, Scotch: Retaliation

Thornapple: Deceitful charms

Thorns, Branch of: Severity

Thrift: Sympathy

Throatwort: Neglected beauty

Thyme: Activity

Tiger Flower: For once may pride befriend me

Traveler's Joy: Safety

Tree of Life: Old age

Trefoil: Revenge

Tremella: Resistance

Trillium Pictum: Modest beauty

Truffle: Surprise

Tulip, Red: Declaration of love

Tulip, Variegated: Beautiful eyes

Tulip, Yellow: Hopeless love

Turnip: Charity

Tussilago, Sweet-scented: Justice shall be done you

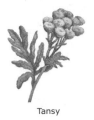

Tansy

V, W

Valerian: An accommodating disposition

Valerian, Greek: Rupture

Venus' Car: Fly with me

Venus' Looking Glass: Flattery

Venus Trap: Deceit

Verbena, Scarlet: Sensibility

Verbena, White: Pure and guileless

Vernal Grass: Poor, but happy

Veronica: Fidelity

Vervain: Enchantment

Vine: Intoxication

Violet, Blue: Faithfulness

Violet, Dame: Watchfulness

Violet, Sweet: Modesty

Violet, Yellow: Rural happiness

Virginia Creeper: Ever changing

Virgin's Bower: Filial love

Volkmannia: May you be happy

Walnut: Intellect, stratagem

Wallflower: Fidelity in adversity

Water Lily: Purity of heart

Wax Plant: Susceptibility

Weigela: Accept a faithful heart

Wheat Stalk: Riches

Whin: Anger

White Lily: Purity and modesty

White Mullein: Good nature

White Oak: Independent

Whortleberry: Treason

Willow, Creeping: Love forsaken

Willow, Water: Freedom

Willow, Weeping: Mourning

Willow, Herb: Pretension

Willow, French: Bravery, humanity

Wisteria: I cling to thee

Witch Hazel: A spell

Woodbine: Fraternal love

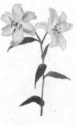

White lily

X, Y, Z

Xanthium: Rudeness, pertinacity

Xeranthemum: Cheerfulness under adversity

Yew: Sorrow

Zephyr Flower: Expectation

Zinnia: Thoughts of absent friends

ABOUT THE AUTHOR

Cerridwen Greenleaf has worked with many of the leading lights of the spirituality world, including Starhawk, Z Budapest, John Michael Greer, Christopher Penczak, Raymond Buckland, Luisah Teish, and many more. She gives herbal workshops throughout North America. Greenleaf's graduate work in medieval studies has given her deep knowledge she utilizes in her recounting of ancient lore, making her work unique in the field. She has sold over 100,000 copies of her books; her latest titles include *The Witch's Guide to Ritual, Moon Spell Magic for Love, The Magic Oracle Book*, and *Mystical Crystals*.

Make sure to check out her inspiring blogs!

- witchesandpagans.com/pagan-culture-blogs/middle-earth-magic.html
- yourmagicalhome.blogspot.com

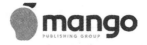

Mango Publishing, established in 2014, publishes an eclectic list of books by diverse authors—both new and established voices—on topics ranging from business, personal growth, women's empowerment, LGBTQ studies, health, and spirituality to history, popular culture, time management, decluttering, lifestyle, mental wellness, aging, and sustainable living. We were recently named 2019 *and* 2020's #1 fastest growing independent publisher by *Publishers Weekly*. Our success is driven by our main goal, which is to publish high quality books that will entertain readers as well as make a positive difference in their lives.

Our readers are our most important resource; we value your input, suggestions, and ideas. We'd love to hear from you—after all, we are publishing books for you!

Please stay in touch with us and follow us at:

Facebook: Mango Publishing
Twitter: @MangoPublishing
Instagram: @MangoPublishing
LinkedIn: Mango Publishing
Pinterest: Mango Publishing
Newsletter: mangopublishinggroup.com/newsletter

Join us on Mango's journey to reinvent publishing, one book at a time.

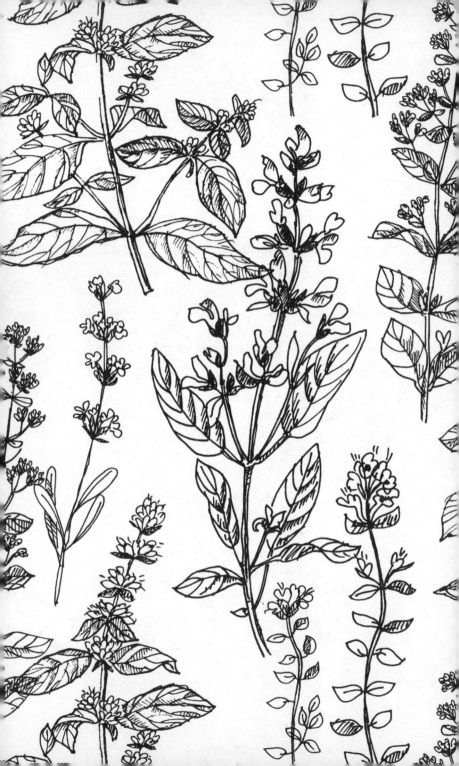